Laboratory Experiences in Exercise Science

Laboratory Experiences in Exercise Science

James D. George
Arizona State University

A. Garth Fisher
Brigham Young University

Pat R. Vehrs
University of Houston

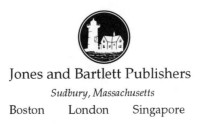

Jones and Bartlett Publishers
Sudbury, Massachusetts
Boston   London   Singapore

Editorial, Sales, and Customer Service Offices
Jones and Bartlett Publishers
40 Tall Pine Drive
Sudbury, MA 01776
(508) 443-5000
(800) 832-0034

Jones and Bartlett Publishers International
Barb House, Barb Mews
London W6 7PA
UK

ISBN: 0-86720-783-3

Acquisitions Editor: Joseph E. Burns
Manufacturing Buyer: Dana L. Cerrito
Design & Typesetting: LeGwin Associates
Editorial Production Service: Colophon
Cover Design: Hannus Design Associates
Printing and Binding: Braun-Brumfield, Inc.
Cover Printing: Phoenix Color Corp.

Printed in the United States of America
98 97 96   10 9 8 7 6 5 4 3

Contents

Preface

This laboratory text is intended for students who are preparing for professions in physical education, exercise science, health promotion, coaching, physical therapy, athletic training, and sports medicine. The primary objective of this text is to provide practical, hands-on experience with tests and measures commonly employed in human performance research laboratories.

Laboratory Experiences in Exercise Science is designed for use in a one-semester, upper-level undergraduate or beginning graduate-level exercise science related course. Because a number of laboratory experiences are offered, instructors are given a large degree of freedom to select the specific materials that correspond to and complement lecture material. In this way, instructors can reinforce basic principles taught in lecture and at the same time allow students to develop basic skills in measurement and evaluation.

This laboratory text utilizes a unique, research-based approach which stimulates students to think and reason intuitively. For instance, each laboratory experience is organized into three basic components: 1) research questions, 2) data collection and determination of results, and 3) research conclusions. The advantage of such an approach is that students not only learn how to collect data (administer tests), but are also given an opportunity to analyze their results and draw their own conclusions.

Our experience over the past several years has taught us that students enjoy the format presented in this laboratory text. A pivotal reason, we believe, for this enjoyment, is that students appreciate the opportunity to apply their knowledge of exercise science to practical, "real life" situations. In addition, we have found that students like an organized approach, one that attempts to minimize confusion and maximize learning outcomes.

We've tried to make this laboratory text as meaningful and useful as possible, and hope that you will find it an invaluable resource. In fact, we would greatly appreciate your comments regarding the effectiveness of this text. As you use it, please make note of any passages that appear unclear or incorrect and also any possible topics that could be incorporated in future editions. We will gladly attempt to implement any suggestions you provide for us.

CONTENTS AND ORGANIZATION

A brief overview of the various laboratory experiences contained in this text is outlined below:

Chapter 1 serves as an introduction and covers fundamental concepts, principles, and terminology discussed in subsequent chapters. Health-related physical fitness, the scientific method, and basic principles of prediction (regression) are presented in Section 1; Section 2 provides a discussion of common terminology encountered in exercise science and the metric system of measurement; and Section 3 outlines valuable information used to screen individuals who wish to perform various physical fitness tests and/or start an exercise program.

Chapters 2, 3, 5, and 6 are designed to address the five components of health-related physical fitness, namely, muscular endurance, flexibility, cardiorespiratory endurance, and body composition. Ample exposure to each component of physical fitness is provided through a variety of meaningful activities. Some of the tests and measures included in these chapters include: a one-repetition maximum bench press, strength-to-weight ratios, a practical muscular strength and endurance test, a grip dynamometer test, a modified sit-and-reach test, four field test used to assess cardiorespiratory endurance, various prediction tests designed to estimate body composition, and hydrostatic weighing.

The measurement of heart rate and blood pressure is described in Chapter 4 and students are expected to evaluate both resting and exercise data. Skills and competencies learned in this chapter are used in several subsequent laboratory experiences.

Chapter 7 gives the student an opportunity to measure overall physical fitness. A variety of test options are available along with the AAHPERD Physical Best program and AFROTC (Air Force ROTC) test battery. The idea of a comprehensive fitness test is valuable since many students, when in their respective professions (i.e., sports medicine clinics, health promotion programs), will be expected to perform such evaluations for their clientele.

Chapter 8 explains basic principles of muscular fatigue and ischemia. A unique laboratory experience is outlined to reinforce fundamental principles related to this topic area.

Chapter 9 provides an opportunity to measure and evaluate anaerobic muscular power. Tests employed within this laboratory experience include the Margaria-Kalamen Power Test and the Wingate Power Test.

Chapter 10 describes various ways to measure and predict resting and exercise energy expenditure and oxygen consumption. The American College of Sports Medicine (ACSM) oxygen cost prediction equations are discussed in detail and students are taught how to effectively apply these equations in a variety of situations.

Chapter 11 provides an introduction to basic electrocardiography. Laboratory activities consist of electrode preparation, measurement of resting and exercise ECGs, and evaluation of results.

Chapter 12 outlines a protocol for the measurement of VO_{2max}. Accordingly, students learn to 1) compute VO_{2max} scores from raw test data, and 2) evaluate this important measure of cardiorespiratory endurance. In addition, basic principles of STPD gas correction are introduced and a variety of meaningful research questions are addressed.

Chapter 13 outlines test protocols for both static and dynamic pulmonary function tests. The static pulmonary measures include the assessment of vital capacity and the three lung volumes associated with this lung capacity (tidal volume, inspiratory reserve volume, and expiratory reserve volume); the dynamic pulmonary function tests include measures of forced expiratory volumes. Residual volume tests are also introduced and BTPS gas correction principles briefly discussed.

Appendixes. The five appendixes consist of 1) Cardiopulmonary Resuscitation, 2) Metric System, 3) Gas Correction Tables and Formula, 4) Sample Problems with Solutions, and 5) Sources for Equipment.

PEDAGOGICAL AIDS
The following pedagogical aids are included in this laboratory text to optimize student learning:

1. At the beginning of each chapter, students are required to complete a Pre-Laboratory Assignment. The purpose for this assignment is to help students understand and become familiar with data collection procedures prior to their scheduled laboratory class period.
2. Each chapter begins with a stated purpose and a list of specific student learning objectives.
3. Numerous computational examples are provided to ensure that students understand how to make necessary calculations.
4. Data sheets are prepared for students so that test results can easily be organized and made ready for evaluation.
5. A listing of selected references are provided for each laboratory experience.
6. Additional sample problems and solutions are outlined in Appendix D.

EQUIPMENT NEEDS
We've tried to develop a variety of laboratory experiences which require only minimal equipment. However, in the event that your laboratory does not have the needed equipment, students can be given reasonable "textbook" data and still be afforded the opportunity to organize and evaluate research conclusions. To aid you in the acquisition of needed equipment, a listing of equipment sources is provided in Appendix E.

ACKNOWLEDGMENTS
We wish to acknowledge and thank the various lab instructors and many students who have helped us evaluate and refine the research-based approach utilized in this laboratory text. Specific thanks are extended to Garth Babcock, Drew Weidman, Dr. Mike Bracko, Patrick Kelly, Donna Winterton, Jeff Peugnet, Deanna Ostergaurd, Dr. Robert Conlee, and Dr. Phil Allsen.

Laboratory Experiences
in Exercise Science

1

Introduction to Exercise Science

1.1
Introduction to Exercise Science and Physical Fitness

PURPOSE
The purpose of this section is to introduce you to the exciting areas of exercise science and physical-fitness assessment.

STUDENT LEARNING OBJECTIVES
1. Be able to describe how the scientific method is used to advance information and knowledge.
2. Be able to outline the basic components of physical fitness and describe how prediction tests are developed to evaluate physical fitness.

EXERCISE SCIENCE
Exercise science encompasses a wide variety of subject areas such as physiology, kinesiology, anatomy, cardiology, endocrinology, bioenergetics, biochemistry, nutrition, and sport psychology. Many professional disciplines utilize various principles of exercise science. A few professions that rely on exercise science include: physical therapy, recreational therapy, cardiac rehabilitation, sports nutrition, health promotion, coaching, dance-related careers, and medical professions.

The American College of Sports Medicine (ACSM) and American Alliance for Health Physical Education Recreation and Dance (AAHPERD) are two prominent organizations that help disseminate new information to professionals in exercise-science related fields. These organizations conduct certification workshops, sponsor regional and national conferences, award research grants, and provide educational materials to both the professional and general public.

Research is an integral part of exercise science. Our current understanding of exercise science is the result of both past and present research. Although not all professionals in exercise science conduct research, those who do so generally focus on either a basic or applied approach.

Basic Scientific Approach
The basic scientific approach examines the underlying scientific foundation of exercise science. The experimental model is often highly technical and tends

to be theoretical in nature. Examples of this type of research might include the study of muscle-fiber type transformations or the metabolic effects of particular drugs.

Applied Scientific Approach

The applied scientific approach, on the other hand, relates the principles of exercise science to practical, real-life situations. The primary purpose of this type of research is often to investigate and disperse information that will enhance athletic performance, improve physical fitness, or prevent disease. Research examples include: studying the effectiveness of various weight control programs, validating new ways to measure physical fitness, and comparing the physiological effects of two aerobic training programs.

Students in the exercise sciences should gain an appreciation of both basic and applied research. Applied research could not exist without basic theoretical research having been conducted. In addition, basic research is of little value unless it can be applied. To become competent in the exercise sciences, a person should have a working knowledge of both areas. Regrettably, some fail to observe this global viewpoint stated by T.H. Huxley in 1948:

> I often wish that this phrase "applied science" had never been invented. For it suggests that there is a sort of scientific knowledge of direct practical use, which can be studied apart from another sort of scientific knowledge, which is of no practical utility, and which is termed "pure science." But there is no more complete fallacy than this. What people call applied science is nothing but the application of pure science to particular classes of problems. It consists of deductions from those principles, established by reasoning and observation, which constitute pure science. No one can safely make these deductions until he has a firm grasp of the principles; and he can obtain that grasp only by personal experience of the operations of observation and of reasoning on which they are found. (Rowell, 1986)

SCIENTIFIC METHOD

The scientific method involves a systematic process for solving problems. The scientific approach consists of the presentation of ideas or questions (hypoth-

Table 1–1
Steps in the Scientific Method

1. Formulation of research question or problem (hypothesis).
2. Collection of relevant data.
3. Formulation of conclusions based on relevant data.

eses), the collection of data or information relevant to the hypotheses, and the approval or denial of the hypotheses based on the evaluation of the relevant data (conclusions) (Table 1–1).

It should be evident that those who systematically analyze their ideas and take appropriate steps to solve their problems are most likely to arrive at legitimate conclusions. In our increasingly complex society, individuals who make the best use of the scientific method will be the most successful scientists, educators, coaches, and health professionals.

A practical application of the scientific method is outlined below:

1. **Research Question**
   How closely does the following regression equation predict maximum heart rate (HR_{max})?

   $$\text{Maximum Heart Rate} = 220 - \text{age}$$

2. **Data Collection**
   a. Select a random sample of individuals, 15 males and 15 females, from each of the following age groups: 10–19 yrs; 20–29 yrs; 30–39 yrs; 40–49 yrs; 50–59 yrs; 60–69 yrs; 70–79 yrs.
   b. Exercise each person to maximum exertion on a treadmill. Measure and record HR_{max} response using ECG equipment.
   c. Based on the data collected, determine the accuracy of the above prediction equation. (Past research has found that the accuracy of this equation for a given person in the population is about ± 15 beats per minute (bpm).)

3. **Discussions/Conclusions**
   a. The above regression equation (220 – age) can predict HR_{max} to within ± 15 bpm. Therefore, a 20-year-old would have a HR_{max} rate between 185 and 215 bpm.
   b. Possible error in the above research could include:

(1) The subjects used in the research may not have represented the entire population and therefore estimates of *actual* variability of HR_{max} across the population was biased.

(2) The ECG equipment may have been inaccurate in the assessment of HR_{max}. If the equipment was inconsistent in heart rate measurement, this may explain the variability of the results.

(3) Some subjects may not have reached a true HR_{max} and consequently increased the variability of the data. This might happen when subjects are not motivated to work to maximum exertion and/or are unaccustomed to running on a treadmill and terminate the test prematurely because of muscle fatigue.

c. Although the regression equation 220−age can predict maximum heart rate, discretion should be used when applying this formulae across the general population. For instance, because this equation is used to determine a heart rate training zone for an exercise program, perhaps the training zone could be expanded to allow for possible prediction error.

PHYSICAL FITNESS

Physical fitness is a set of attributes that enables one to successfully meet the present and potential physical challenges of daily life. Physical challenges may be imposed by work, daily routines, exercise, and emergency situations. Physical fitness is often viewed as a continuum. The upper end of the spectrum includes individuals who can carry out daily tasks with vigor and alertness, with ample energy to enjoy leisure-time activities and meet unforeseen emergencies. The lower end of the spectrum includes individuals who have a diminished ability to meet even the lowest of physical demands and may be completely dependent on others to survive.

There are five health-related components of physical fitness:

1. Muscular strength
2. Muscular endurance
3. Cardiorespiratory endurance
4. Joint range of motion; flexibility
5. Body composition (fat-to-lean ratio)

Acceptable levels of physical fitness should be achieved for each of the five components. However, some individuals may possess an adequate level of physical fitness in one component and inadequate levels in others. For example, a football athlete who plays on the offensive line may be very strong, yet have excess body fat and low cardiorespiratory endurance. Fortunately the health-related aspects of physical fitness are modifiable and can be improved with regular physical activity and good nutrition.

PHYSICAL FITNESS TESTS

There are several reasons why individuals should have their physical fitness evaluated. For example:

1. The health-related components of physical fitness that need improvement can be clearly determined.
2. Realistic and meaningful goals can be set to improve and/or maintain particular components of physical fitness.
3. Safe and effective training regimens can be designed based on the results of a fitness evaluation.
4. Baseline levels of fitness can be established upon which to chart progress and monitor improvement.
5. Fitness evaluations may enhance motivation and help individuals stay with their fitness program.

To evaluate physical fitness, appropriate tests must be available. Generally two types of tests are used to measure physical fitness—standard tests and prediction tests.

Standard tests These are considered by exercise scientists as the preferred method of testing since such tests are the most valid, reliable, and precise.

Advantage: Provide relatively accurate measures of physical fitness.

Disadvantages: Often require expensive equipment, trained personnel, and a significant time commitment for both the test administrator and subject.

Prediction tests These tests are designed to indirectly estimate or predict physical fitness. Prediction tests are usually correlated to standard tests and serve to estimate the results of a standard test.

Table 1–2
Health-Related Physical Fitness Tests

Fitness Parameter	Standard Test	Prediction Test
Muscular strength	Isokinetic measures 1 repetition max	Hand-grip dynamometer
Muscular endurance	Isokinetic measures Endurance tests	1 Minute sit-up test
Joint flexibility	Goniometer measures Leighton flexometer	Sit and reach test
Cardiorespiratory endurance	Treadmill VO_{2max}	Astrand cycle test 1.5-mile run 1.0-mile jog Step test
Body composition	Hydrodensitometry	Skin folds Girth measurements

Advantages: Relatively inexpensive, require minimal equipment, easily administered, and allow for testing of large groups of people at one time.

Disadvantage: Less accurate than standard tests.

A summary of common standard and prediction tests used to evaluate health-related physical fitness are outlined in Table 1–2.

Because of the practical limitations associated with standard tests, researchers often devise prediction tests. It is important to understand how prediction tests are developed. Let's say that we want to develop a new method to predict percent body fat. From our observations we notice that lean individuals have a thin subcutaneous fat layer and that obese individuals have a thick subcutaneous fat layer. We wonder if the observed relationship could allow us to accurately predict total body fat and thereby provide a less expensive and more convenient test than traditional hydrostatic (underwater) weighing.

We decide to organize a research project and test our hypothesis. First, we advertise in the local paper and recruit 50 male and 50 female subjects, ranging from 20 to 70 years of age. In so doing, we select subjects with a wide range of body fat levels. We know that to develop an accurate, representative prediction equation for the general population we need subjects who possess differing levels of body fat.

Each subject is asked to come to our laboratory and be measured with both the hydrostatic weighing technique (standard) and new skin fold technique. Accordingly, the percent fat of each subject is determined with the hydrostatic technique. In addition, various skin-fold measurements are recorded. After all 100 subjects are tested, the data are statistically analyzed to determine whether a meaningful relationship between hydrostatic measurement of body fat and subcutaneous fat measurements is present.

Based on the data, we plot the relationship between hydrostatic percent fat and sum of skin fold measurements (Figure 1–1). From this plot, you see that a positive linear relationship exists between these variables. You should also realize that each data point on the graph represents a given subject's hydrostatic weighing percent fat. This means that for any sum of skin fold measurement along the x axis, each data point is positioned in reference to the y axis (i.e., % fat from the hydrostatic weighing test). For instance, if a subject's sum of skin fold measurement is 60 mm and she is hydrostatically weighed at 38% fat, then the data point on the graph will be positioned above the 60 mm mark on the x axis and across from the 38% fat mark on the y axis. Likewise, if a subject's sum of skin fold measurement is 40 mm and he was hydrostatically weighed at 20% fat, then the data point on the graph will be positioned above the 40 mm mark on the x axis and across from the 20% fat mark on the y axis. Understanding this logic will help you see how skin fold measurements are used to predict hydrostatic percent fat results.

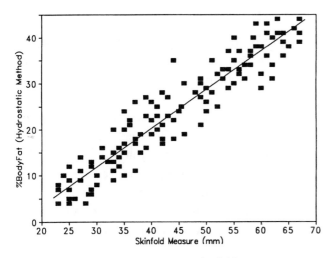

Figure 1–1 Plot of Hydrostatic vs. Skinfold Data.

Notice that a line has been drawn through the middle of the data points in Figure 1–1. This line is called the *line of best fit* because it is placed in an average position, with approximately half of the data points above the line and half the data points below the line. This line represents the average hydrostatic weighing results of both the male and female subjects, as generated from their skin fold measurements.

Once a line of best fit is properly set in place, it can be used to predict outcomes for individuals who were not a part of the original research study. This means that someone could have a percent fat estimate of hydrostatic weighing without actually performing the test. For example, if a subject was measured to have a sum of skin folds of 30 mm, one would first draw a vertical line up from the x axis to the line of best fit and then draw a horizontal line over to the y axis to *predict* hydrostatic results of ≈12%. Thus, the line of best fit serves as a prediction line.

The line of best fit is also commonly called a regression line because it can be used to generate a mathematical equation called a *regression equation*. A regression equation is based on the simple mathematical equation $y = mx + b$ assuming a linear (straight) regression line is used. You may recall from a basic math class that m represents the slope of the line; x represents numbers along the x axis; b represents the y axis intercept; and y represents numbers along the y axis.

Suppose the regression equation for the line of best fit in Figure 1–1 is:

$$y = 0.51x + 4.5$$

In this case, the x value represents the sum of skin fold measurements and the y value represents estimated hydrostatic weighing measurements. Accordingly, the above regression equation could enable one to insert x values into the equation and solve for y. What then, would be the estimated hydrostatic weighing percent fat of a person who had a sum of skin fold measurement of 50 mm? (Insert 50 into the equation and solve for y.)

$$0.51(50) + 4.5 = 30\%$$

Thus, the above regression equation estimates what an individual's percent body fat would be if they had actually performed the hydrostatic weighing test.

Can you see how the above regression equation could be made more accurate? Include other variables (i.e., gender, age) in the regression equation which may help predict more accurate hydrostatic weighing percent fat scores. In addition, the regression equation could be tested (cross-validated) on various other samples to determine its generalizability across the population.

One way to assess the accuracy of a prediction test is to consider a quantitative measure called a *correlation coefficient* or *r-value*. A high correlation, $r = \pm 0.90$ to 0.99, generally indicates that data points closely surround the line of best fit. Conversely, a lower correlation, $r = \pm 0.60$ to 0.80, generally reflects data points spread more widely above and below the line of best fit.

A second way to assess the accuracy of a prediction test is to consider what is called the *standard error of estimate* (SEE). The SEE, like the r-value, is based on the degree of spread surrounding the line of best fit. However, the SEE provides a meaningful estimate of how well a given prediction test can estimate the results of the standard test. For example, research generally demonstrates that the skinfold test has a SEE of ± 3.7 percent body fat. This means that if a skinfold regression equation predicts a percent fat of 15, then the actual hydrostatic weighing percent fat would likely be between 11.3 and 18.7 percent fat, 68 percent of the time.

The practical value of a regression equation depends on its accuracy. To maximize the usefulness of a particular prediction test all possible error must be minimized. Outlined below are suggestions that may help to limit the error associated with prediction tests.

1. Use regression (prediction) equations derived from

a sample that most closely parallels the subject's characteristics (i.e., age, gender, fitness level, etc.).

2. Be sure to perform the prediction test exactly as it was performed in the original research.

3. Select a prediction test that is most appropriate for a particular subject. For example, the 1.5-mile run to estimate cardiorespiratory endurance would not be an appropriate test for evaluating a sedentary adult.

4. Be sure that test administrators are skilled and know the difference between usual and unusual test results. Also be confident that participants understand how to prepare for and perform test protocols.

5. Verify that all equipment is calibrated correctly and working properly and that the environment (air temperature and humidity) is comfortable for the participant .

The above discussion is vital and should help you understand the difference between standard tests and prediction tests. Accordingly, you should realize that prediction methods are never more accurate than standard methods, assuming both methods are performed according to protocol, and that prediction tests have inherent error that must be minimized.

1.2
Common Terminology and
the Metric System of Measurement

PURPOSE
The purpose of this section is to review common terminology encountered in exercise science and provide a brief introduction to the metric system of measurement.

STUDENT LEARNING OBJECTIVES
1. Be able to understand common terminology used in exercise science.
2. Have a workable understanding of the metric system of measurement.
3. Be familiar with standard unit values of frequently measured parameters and demonstrate the ability to convert from one unit value to another.

TERMINOLOGY
To understand current research and laboratory experiences, a knowledge of frequently used terms is imperative. Experts in the area of exercise science as well as the American College of Sports Medicine (ACSM) have provided definitions of terms to promote consistency and clarity of communication. Some of these terms and definitions are listed below.

Physical Activity   Any bodily movement produced by skeletal muscles that results in energy expenditure

Exercise   A subset of physical activity that is planned, structured, and repetitive and has as a final or an intermediate objective the improvement or maintenance of physical fitness

Exercise Intensity   A specific level of maintenance of muscular activity that can be quantified

Endurance   The time period for which a person can maintain a specific isometric force or a specific power level involving combinations of concentric or eccentric muscular contractions

Energy   The capability of producing force, performing work, or generating heat, expressed in joules or kilojoules

Force   That which changes the state of rest or motion in matter, expressed in newtons

Power   The rate of performing work. The product of force and velocity (distance divided by time), expressed in watts

Speed   The total distance traveled per unit time, expressed as meters-per-second

Work   Force applied through a distance but with no limitation on time, expressed as joules or kilojoules

Volume   An occupied or unoccupied space expressed in liters or milliliters

The following terms are also frequently used in exercise science:

Per   Indicates a function of division. For example, 5

liters-per-minute denotes that the total number of liters is divided by the total number of minutes, i.e., 25 liters ÷ 5 minutes = 5 liters-per-min.

Percent Means *per hundred* or *portion of the whole*. For instance, percent fat is a relative value that reflects how much fat there is on a body in proportion to the total mass. A person weighing 100 pounds of which 20 pounds are fat would be 20% fat (20 pounds ÷ 100 pounds). Likewise a person weighing 180 pounds of which 36 pounds are fat would also be 20% fat. The usage of percents and percentages has various applications. For example, if a subject in a lab was lifting 23 pounds, and her one-repetition maximum (1 RM) is 46 pounds, then this person would be working at 50% of maximum strength.

Rate In exercise science, rate indicates a time frame for a given test parameter. In other words, the quantity is expressed as a measurement per unit time. For example, in exercise science the rate of oxygen consumption is often expressed as the amount of oxygen consumed per minute (i.e., 0.25 liters/minute).

Mean Is synonymous with *average*. A mean or average can be computed by summing all observations and dividing by the total number of observations. For example, if we observed the following resting heart rates of 67, 65, 72, 62, 70, 68, and 66, we could compute the mean as follows:

$$\text{Mean} = \frac{67 + 65 + 72 + 62 + 70 + 68 + 66}{7}$$
$$= 67.14 \text{ beats/min.}$$

Valid *Valid* implies that a given test measures the parameter of interest. If percent body fat is the parameter of interest, then a test that measures or accurately estimates body fat is considered a valid test. Whether or not a test is valid can be determined by understanding a test's theoretical basis and by conducting research to confirm such theories and beliefs.

Reliable Means that a given test will provide consistent results on successive measures. In order for reliability to be high, all sources of measurement error must be minimized. *Caution:* A prediction test may have good test/retest reliability yet have a very large SEE and therefore be invalid. For example, if body weight is used to predict the re-

sults of hydrostatic weighing, body weight measures might be very reliable, yet be very inadequate in the prediction of percent fat. Tests can therefore be reliable and not valid.

Objectivity Represents the ability of a test to give similar results when administered by different administrators. Objectivity is also referred to as inter-observer reliability.

Absolute Although there are various definitions of the term, we will use the following: *Absolute* means that the measurement in question is specific to the individual or thing. In other words, the value is unrelated to and independent of anyone or anything else. A common absolute measure used in exercise science is maximal oxygen consumption (VO_{2max}) expressed in $L \cdot min^{-1}$.

Relative Means that a given measurement relates in some way to other measurements. Relative measures provide a means of comparison since measurements can be ranked and categorized. An example of a relative measure is VO_{2max} expressed in $ml \cdot kg^{-1} \cdot min^{-1}$ since test results can be compared across individuals with differing body weights. Without relative or comparative measures, many exercise physiology measurements have little meaning for the general population.

Norms Norm charts describe or rank an individual's measured score. Typically, norm charts rank an individual according to categories (i.e., poor, good, excellent, etc.). Norm charts are derived from research involving large groups of people and the ranking scheme is based on percentile computations. A typical ranking scheme rates scores into one of five categories: poor, fair, average, good, and excellent. For example, twenty percent of the population with the lowest scores could be used to define the poor category. The fair, average, and good categories could be represented within the 20th to 40th, 40th to 60th, and 60th to 80th percentiles, respectively. Scores above the 80th percentile could represent an excellent rating.

METRIC SYSTEM OF MEASUREMENT

The metric system has been accepted as the standard unit of measure in many scientific fields. The metric system has replaced the Imperial system of measurement which uses different measures to quantify volume (cup, pint, quart, gallon), length (inch, foot, yard, mile), and weight (pound, tons).

The nomenclature used for the metric system is the International System of Units (abbreviated SI from the French term *Systeme International*). There is only one standard measurement for a given parameter, such as weight, volume or length. All other measurements of a given parameter are related to the standard measurement and to each other by factors of 10. Larger or smaller measurements are merely recorded as a decimal of the base unit. For example, the standard unit of measure for length is the meter. Lengths shorter than a meter can be recorded as a decimal of a meter.

Rather than use decimals all of the time, prefixes are used to denote a fraction or multiple of the base unit. Prefixes are an important part of understanding the metric system.

kilo (k) = 1000 = 10^3
hecto (h) = 100 = 10^2
deka (da) = 10 = 10^1
deci (d) = 0.1 = 10^{-1}
centi (c) = 0.01 = 10^{-2}
milli (m) = 0.001 = 10^{-3}

- VOLUME: Basic unit of measure is the liter (L).

  1 liter = 10 dL = 100 cL = 1000 mL

- WEIGHT: Basic unit of measure is the gram (g).

  1 gram = 10 dg = 100 cg = 1000 mg
  1 kilogram = 1000 grams = 1,000,000 mg

- LENGTH: Basic unit of measure is the meter (m).

  1 meter = 10 dm = 100 cm = 1000 mm

Always write down the correct unit value (i.e., gm, m, mL) that goes along with each numerical value. When recording data in tables, unit values are often written at the head of each column and therefore it is unnecessary to write the unit value for each entry. Refer to Appendix B for further information about proper expression of data.

Since the metric system is the accepted system of reporting data it is necessary to be able to convert measured values from Imperial units into metric units. You must also be able to convert metric values into smaller or larger unit values. A few standard conversion factors (metric equivalents) include:

1 kg = 2.205 pounds
1 lb = 0.4536 kg
1 inch = 2.54 centimeters

For example, if a male weighs 220 lbs, what is his weight in kilograms?

$$22 \text{ lbs} \times \frac{0.4536 \text{ kg}}{1 \text{ lb}} = 99.79 \text{ kg}$$

If a person measures 6 feet tall, how many centimeters does this equal?

$$6 \text{ feet} \times \frac{12 \text{ inches}}{1 \text{ foot}} \times \frac{2.54 \text{ cm}}{1 \text{ inch}} = 182.8 \text{ cm or } 183 \text{ cm}$$

Convert the person's height from centimeters to meters.

$$183 \text{ cm} \times \frac{1 \text{ meter}}{100 \text{ cm}} = 1.83 \text{ meters}$$

Each conversion factor or metric equivalent you use should be written so that the appropriate units can be *cancelled* from the equation. An easy way to do this is to write the initial value at the far left of the equation (220 lbs) and then position the appropriate equivalent with the units you wish to cancel out as the denominator (1 lb). See the first example above. Now multiply the initial value by your equivalent to cancel out the proper units (pounds). You are left with the desired units in kilograms. A reversal of this process is to convert 99.79 kg into pounds. Such would be written:

$$99.79 \text{ kg} \times \frac{1 \text{ lb}}{0.4536 \text{ kg}} = 220 \text{ lbs}$$

Sometimes unit conversions are a bit more tricky. For instance, suppose you wanted to determine the pace in minutes-per-mile of a person who maintained a jogging speed of 5 miles-per-hour. How do you proceed? The first step is to study the unit values and realize that you need to make use of the equivalent 1 hr = 60 min. The next step is to decide how to arrange the equation so as to cancel out the appropriate units. For example:

$$\frac{1 \text{ hr}}{5 \text{ miles}} \times \frac{60 \text{ minutes}}{1 \text{ hr}} = 12.0 \text{ minutes per mile}$$

An alternative equation uses division:

$$\frac{60 \text{ minutes}}{1 \text{ hr}} \div \frac{5.0 \text{ miles}}{1 \text{ hr}} = 12.0 \text{ minutes per mile}$$

Note that the "1 hr" units are cancelled in both examples and we are left with the desired units for our answer.

Be sure that your answers make good, logical sense. Obviously if you computed that the above jogger took 0.833 minutes to run a mile you should quickly realize that this doesn't make sense. Don't simply trust your calculator—always think about your answer and be sure it is logical. In addition, always write down the unit values for each step of a given calculation and cancel appropriate unit values as you complete the problem.

An important question is: How many decimal places should be used to express a given numerical answer? For example, should a percent body fat value be expressed as 10.32% or 10.3239%? The answer depends on both the precision of the device used to make the measurement and the interpretation of the number. Clearly, body fat should be expressed with only two decimal places since equipment used to measure body fat is not precise beyond the second decimal place and a meaningful alteration in body fat usually requires a change of 1–2% body fat. If someone altered his body fat percentage by 0.0032% his athletic performance would not be enhanced nor his risk for disease modified.

Another measure related to body fat assessment, however, requires the use of four decimal places.

Body density values are expressed as 0.9986, not 0.99. The rationale for this is that a body density of 0.9986 corresponds to a percent body fat of 45.69%, while a body density of 0.99 equals 50% body fat. Clearly, very small changes in body density have a profound effect on percent fat computations and, therefore, more decimal places must be utilized. Throughout this manual, with the exception of a few computations (i.e., body density) which require more than two decimal places, numerical values used to describe the components of physical fitness can all be expressed with no more than two decimal places.

Another important issue is when and how to *round* numbers during a series of computations. For instance, should you round the number 54.9278 up to 55.0 for a given computation? Again this depends. If done in the middle of a series of computations, rounding could significantly change the final number (i.e., $55.0 \times 25 = 1375$, $54.9278 \times 25 = 1373.195$); consequently do not round numbers in the middle of a problem. However, a final answer can be rounded. For example, if 54.9278 is the final answer, express the answer as 54.93 or 55.0 depending on the number of decimal places that should be used.

1.3
Pre-Participation Screening

PURPOSE
The purpose of this section is to explain the importance and need for pre-exercise screening evaluations.

STUDENT LEARNING OBJECTIVES
1. Be able to describe the need and purpose for pre-exercise screening.
2. Be able to evaluate the results of pre-exercise screening.

Cardiovascular disease is the number one cause of death in the United States as well as many other developed countries. Sudden death can occur as a result of exercise. Reported deaths during vigorous exercise have been approximated at 1 death per year for every 15,000 to 20,000 people. Obviously regular physical activity does not immunize individuals from death during exercise; however, active individuals do have a significantly lower overall risk of death than sedentary (inactive) individuals.

Many Americans lead sedentary lifestyles and may be at high risk for a number of diseases which can affect their ability to exercise. Because many individuals decide to begin an exercise program at one time or another, there is a need to identify individuals who have an increased risk of medical complications. Although moderate intensity exercise (40 to 60% VO_{2max}) is safe for most individuals, it is suggested that certain individuals have at least a limited health and risk evaluation prior to exercise or exercise testing.

The health status of an individual can be classified as apparently healthy, at high risk for disease, or diseased. The purpose of pre-exercise screening is to ensure the safety of exercise testing and subsequent exercise programs, determine appropriate type(s) of exercise tests or exercise programs, identify individuals in need of more comprehensive evaluations, and identify individuals who may have special needs (i.e., the elderly, pregnant women, diabetics).

Apparently healthy individuals are those who are asymptomatic (without symptoms) with no more than one major coronary risk factor (see Table 1–3). Individuals at higher risk are those who have symptoms (see Table 1–4) suggestive of possible cardiopulmonary or metabolic diseases and/or demonstrate two or more major risk factors of coronary heart disease. Individuals classified as diseased are those with diagnosed cardiac, pulmonary, or metabolic disease.

Men under the age of 40 and women under the age of 50 who are apparently healthy can participate in moderate and vigorous exercise without a pre-par-

Table 1–3
Major Coronary Risk Factors

1. Diagnosed hypertension or systolic blood pressure ≥ 160 or diastolic blood pressure ≥ 90 mmHg on at least two separate occasions, or on antihypertensive medication

2. Serum cholesterol levels ≥ 6.20 mmol/L (≥ 240 mg/dL)

3. Cigarette smoking

4. Diabetes Mellitus.*

5. Family history of coronary or other atherosclerotic disease in patients or siblings prior to age 55.

*Persons with insulin dependent diabetes mellitus (IDDM) who are over 30 years of age, or have had IDDM for more than 15 years, and persons with non-insulin dependent diabetes (NIDDM) who are over 35 years of age should be classified as patients with disease.

From *Guidelines for Exercise Testing and Prescription*, 4th edition, American College of Sports Medicine, Lea & Febiger, 1991.

Table 1–4
Major Symptoms or Signs Suggestive of Cardiopulmonary or Metabolic Disease*

1. Pain or discomfort in the chest or surrounding areas that appears to be ischemic in nature

2. Unaccustomed shortness of breath or shortness of breath with mild exertion

3. Dizziness or syncope

4. Orthopnea/paroxysmal nocturnal dyspnea

5. Ankle edema

6. Palpitations or tachycardia

7. Claudication

8. Known heart murmur

* These symptoms must be interpreted in the clinical context in which they appear since they are not all specific for cardiopulmonary or metabolic disease.
From *Guidelines for Exercise Testing and Prescription*, 4th edition, American College of Sports Medicine, Lea & Febiger, 1991.

ticipation medical exam or diagnostic exercise test. In addition, these individuals can undergo submaximal or maximal exercise tests without the supervision of a physician. However the test should be supervised by trained personnel. For apparently healthy males over 40-years old and apparently healthy females over 50-years-old, a physician must be present for maximal exercise tests but not necessarily for submaximal tests. These older individuals do not require a medical

exam or diagnostic exercise test before participation in moderate intensity exercise (40 to 60% VO_{2max}) but should have such a test prior to vigorous exercise (>60% VO_{2max}).

Asymptomatic individuals at higher risk can participate in moderate but not vigorous intensity exercise without appropriate medical exams or diagnostic exercise test. High-risk individuals with symptoms or individuals with known disease must have a medical exam and diagnostic exercise test prior to participation in any type of exercise. A diagnostic exercise test is one in which workloads are increased until subjects reach volitional fatigue or are limited by symptoms. The volume of oxygen consumed (VO_2) by the subject may or may not be measured, depending on the purpose(s) of the test. Subjects are monitored with an electrocardiogram (ECG or EKG) to observe the electrical activity of the heart as exercise demands increase. Blood pressure is also monitored as are observable signs and symptoms. Based on ECG results, blood pressure responses, and specific signs and symptoms, the attending physicians are able to determine the likelihood of disease. A positive test indicates disease and generally requires (at the physicians discretion) further testing prior to beginning an exercise program. A negative test indicates little likelihood of disease and permits the individual to begin an exercise program.

Regardless of the health or fitness status of an individual, a pre-participation questionnaire should be used to screen for the presence of disease or symptoms suggestive of disease. Pre-participation screening may include personal and medical histories or a Physical Activity Readiness Questionnaire (PAR-Q). The PAR-Q has been suggested as a minimum pre-participation questionnaire. If an individual answers affirmative to any question on the PAR-Q, the person should seek medical counsel and postpone vigorous physical activity and/or exercise testing. Accordingly, all pre-participation screenings must be done with professionalism, wisdom, and prudence.

A medical examination is often recommended for all older adults, even the apparently healthy. As discussed earlier, a diagnostic exercise test may be included in this examination. When a physician suspects advanced cardiovascular disease, the individual will likely be encouraged to undergo further clinical testing such as echocardiography, thallium imaging, or coronary angiography.

INFORMED CONSENT

Prior to exercise testing, individuals should provide written, informed consent to help ensure that all testing procedures, risks, and benefits are completely understood. An informed consent should communicate to the participant that any questions regarding exercise testing are welcomed, withdrawal from participation at any time is allowed, and all information about the participant will be held confidential. A sample of a PAR-Q, personal history questionnaire, and informed consent form are provided as a part of this laboratory experience.

If by answering the screening questionnaires in the following assignment you are identified as being at risk, it is your responsibility to obtain medical clearance from a qualified physician before participation in this laboratory experience.

SELECTED REFERENCES FOR CHAPTER 1

Adams, G. M. *Exercise Physiology Lab Manual* (1990). Dubuque, Iowa: Wm. C. Brown Publishers, pp: 1–17.

American College of Sports Medicine (1991). *Guidelines of Exercise Testing and Prescription* (4th edition). Philadelphia: Lea & Febiger, pp: 1–10, 35–39.

Baumgartner, T. A., and A. S. Jackson (1991). *Measurement for Evaluation in Physical Education and Exercise Science.* Dubuque, Iowa: Wm. C. Brown Publishers.

Brooks, G.A., and T. D. Fahey (1984). *Exercise Physiology: Human Bioenergetics and Its Applications.* New York: John Wiley & Sons, pp: 1–16.

Caspersen, C. J., K. E. Powell, and G. M. Christenson (1985). Physical activity, exercise, and physical fitness: definitions and distinctions for health-related research. *Public Health Reports* March–April: 126–131.

DeVries, H. A. (1986). *Physiology of Exercise: For Physical Education and Athletics* (4th edition). Dubuque, Iowa: Wm. C. Brown Publishers, pp: 5–10, 256–266, 577–578

Fisher, A. G., and C. R. Jensen (1990). *Scientific Basis of Athletic Conditioning* (3rd edition). Philadelphia: Lea & Febiger.

Fox, E. L., R. W. Bowers, and M. L. Foss (1988). *Physiological Basis of Physical Education and Athletics* (4th edition). Philadelphia: Saunders College Publishing, pp: 1–3.

Heyward, V. H., (1991). *Advanced Fitness Assessment and Exercise Prescription.* Champaign, Illinois: Human Kinetics, pp: 1–15.

Hoeger, W. W. K. (1989). *Lifetime Physical Fitness and Wellness: A Personalized Program.* Englewood, Colorado: Morton Publishing Company, pp: 1–13.

Howley, E. T., and D. B. Frank (1992). *Health Fitness Instructor's Handbook* (2nd edition). Champaign, Illinois: Human Kinetics, pp: 3–25, 83–92.

Knuttgen, H.G. (1986 December). Quantifying Exercise Performance with SI Units. *Physician and Sports Medicine* 157–161.

Lamb, D. R. (1984). *Physiology of Exercise: Responses and Adaptations* (2nd edition). New York: Macmillan Publishing Company, pp: 1–9, 366–368.

McArdle, W. D., F. I. Katch, and V. L. Katch (1991). *Exercise Physiology: Energy, Nutrition, and Human Performance* (3rd edition). Philadelphia: Lea & Febiger.

Noble, B. J. (1986). *Physiology of Exercise and Sport.* St. Louis, Missouri: Times Mirror/Mosby College Publishing.

Powers, S. K., and E. T. Howley (1990). *Exercise Physiology: Theory and Application to Fitness and Performance.* Dubuque, Iowa: Wm. C. Brown Publishers, pp: 3–14, 292–302, 305–308, 330–331.

Rowell, L. B. (1986). *Human Circulation: Regulation During Physical Stress.* New York: Oxford University Press.

Wilmore, J. H., and D. L. Costill (1988). *Training for Sport and Activity: The Physiological Basis of the Conditioning Process* (3rd edition). Dubuque, Iowa: Wm. C. Brown Publishers, pp: 361–367.

Young, D.S. (1987). Implementation of SI units for clinical laboratory data. *Annals of Internal Medicine* 106 1:114–129.

Chart 1–3
Informed Consent

As part of this laboratory experience, I understand that I will be asked to perform various tests to evaluate my level of physical fitness. I understand these tests will be administered by myself and/or other students in the class. I am also aware that the administration and performance of such tests are designed to be an educational experience.

I understand that I am free to ask any questions about any test performed in my laboratory class. If for any reason I am unable to perform a given test, I will inform my laboratory instructor. Likewise, if I am unable to administer any test, I will inform my instructor.

There are certain risks associated with any physical fitness evaluation. These include abnormal blood pressure or heart rate responses, heart beat disorders, fainting, and, in rare cases, heart attack, stroke, or death. Every effort will be made to minimize these risks by evaluation of preliminary information relating to my health status and by observation of symptoms during exercise tests.

Because my health status can directly affect my safety during exercise, I will disclose any problems about my health status to my laboratory instructor. I will also promptly report any feelings of discomfort or pain associated with a given test to student associates or my laboratory instructor.

Throughout this laboratory experience, I will be required to share my test results with other class members. However, information about me will not be disclosed to anyone outside of class without my written permission.

My enrollment and consent to participate in this laboratory experience is voluntary and I realize that I am free to withdraw from any test, at any time, for health reasons. If I have any further questions regarding this laboratory experience I am free to contact ___Dr. Odland___ (laboratory director) at this phone number:___395 - 7695___ and/or_____ (department chair) at this phone number:_____.

I have read this form and give written consent to participate in this laboratory experience.

Anne E. Schrah Date:_1/8/98_
Signature of Student

_____
Signature of Witness

Please photocopy and retain a copy for yourself.

2
Muscular Fitness
· ·
Pre-Laboratory Assignment

1. Describe various benefits of muscular fitness.

2. Describe the difference between muscular strength and muscular endurance.

3. Describe at least two factors that affect muscular strength and at least two factors that affect muscular endurance.

4. What is the strength-to-weight ratio of someone with a 1 RM of 105 kg and a body weight of 170 lbs? Show your work.

5. Calculate your exercise weight for Station 3 (page 39) based on the appropriate percent of your body weight. Record your computations.

    Two Arm Curl: _____lbs

    Leg Extension: _____lbs

    Lat Pulldown: _____lbs

    Bench Press: _____lbs

    Leg Curl: _____lbs

6. ❑ Check the box if you have read each research question for this lab and are familiar with the data-collection procedures regarding each research question.

2

Muscular Fitness

Muscular fitness is an important part of overall physical fitness because it promotes good posture and joint integrity, decreases the risk of injury, increases one's functional ability to perform in athletic and recreational events, and helps individuals maintain proper body composition. It may also improve self-esteem.

MUSCULAR STRENGTH

Muscular strength is defined as the ability of the muscular system to exert external force or oppose a given resistance. Muscular strength is often evaluated by a one-repetition maximum (1 RM) which is the maximum amount of weight that can be lifted one time. Strength can also be evaluated with a relative measure such as a strength-to-weight ratio, calculated by dividing strength by body weight.

There are several factors that can affect muscular strength including: the size of the recruited muscle cell (fiber), the size of the recruited motor unit, the number of motor units recruited, the frequency of stimulation, the degree of neuromuscular inhibition, energy stores (ATP-PC and glycogen), internal temperature levels, and waste-product accumulation.

In essence, the more myosin cross-bridges cycling at a given moment, the greater the generation of muscular force. Thus, if a person can recruit large motor units with large muscle fibers, stimulate the muscle with optimal excitation, and provide a proper cellular environment with accompanying fuel stores, muscular force will be at a maximal level.

Other factors that may affect strength (force generation) include: mechanical factors such as muscle fiber length, speed of contraction, joint angle, lever arm relationships; skill and lifting technique; the type of muscular contraction performed—eccentric versus concentric; and the ability of bone, connective tissue, and supporting structures to withstand the stress of the lift.

MUSCULAR ENDURANCE

Muscular endurance is the ability of the muscular system to exert external force or oppose a resistance for a given number of repetitions and/or for a given period of time. Muscular endurance can be expressed in absolute or relative terms. Absolute endurance infers that a person can lift a given weight a prescribed number of repetitions and/or for a period of time. Relative endurance, on the other hand, expresses muscular endurance in terms of the percent of an individual's maximum ability. For example, John's 1 RM bicep curl was 80 pounds and Bill's 1 RM curl was 100 pounds. Both attempted to curl 50 pounds as many times as possible. Even though they were both lifting the same absolute weight (50 pounds), John lifted 65% of his 1 RM and Bill lifted only 50% of his 1 RM.

Muscular endurance is influenced by many of the same factors that influence muscular strength (i.e., number of recruited motor units, energy stores, etc.). Research has demonstrated that muscular endurance is highly correlated to muscular strength. Unlike muscular strength, however, muscular endurance is additionally influenced by the amount of blood circulated through the active muscle.

Note: Blood flow to and from muscle is significantly reduced when the workout is above 60 to 70% of maximum strength (% 1 RM). One reason for this is that during intense muscular contractions, blood vessels are compressed by skeletal muscle and occluded. Because energy demands are higher and blood flow reduced, muscular endurance can be greatly hindered during high intensity resistive exercise. Accordingly it may be of value to consider the intensity (% 1 RM) of the exercise when endurance is measured.

SELECTED REFERENCES

Adams, G. M. *Exercise Physiology Lab Manual* (1990). Dubuque, Iowa: Wm. C. Brown Publishers, pp: 171–183.

American College of Sports Medicine (1991). *Guidelines of Exercise Testing and Prescription* (4th edition). Philadelphia: Lea & Febiger, pp: 48–54.

DeVries, H. A. (1986). *Physiology of Exercise: For Physical Education and Athletics* (4th edition). Dubuque, Iowa: Wm. C. Brown Publishers, pp: 17–20, 57–62, 398–409, 412–420, 442–459.

Fisher, A. G., and C. R. Jensen (1991). *Scientific Basis of Athletic Conditioning* (3rd edition). Philadelphia: Lea & Febiger, pp: 19–23, 139–160.

Fitness Canada (1987). *Canadian Standardized Test of Fitness: Operations Manual.* (3rd edition). Ottawa, Canada: Fitness and Amateur Sports Directorate.

Fox, E. L., R. W. Bowers, and M. L. Foss (1988). *The Physiological Basis of Physical Education and Athletics* (4th edition). Philadelphia: Saunders College Publishing, pp: 100–133, 158–166.

Heyward, V. H. (1991). *Advanced Fitness Assessment and Exercise Prescription.* Champaign, Illinois: Human Kinetic Books, pp: 99–117.

Hoeger, W.W.K. (1991). *Principles and Labs for Physical Fitness and Wellness.* Englewood, Colorado: Morton Publishing.

Hoeger, W. W. K. (1989). *Lifetime Physical Fitness and Wellness: A Personalized Program.* Englewood, Colorado: Morton Publishing Company, pp: 43–79.

Hoeger, W.W.K., S. L. Barette, D. F. Hale, and D. R. Hopkins (1987). Relationship between repetitions and selected percentages of one repetition maximum. *Journal of Applied Sport Science Research* 1(1):11–13.

Howley, E. T., and D. B. Frank (1992). *Health Fitness Instructor's Handbook* (2nd edition). Champaign, Illinois: Human Kinetics, pp: 32–35, 179–184.

Jackson, A., M. Watkins, and R. Patton (1980). A factor analysis of twelve selected maximal isotonic strength performances on the Universal Gym. *Medicine and Science in Sport and Exercise* 12:274–277.

Lamb, D. R. (1984). *Physiology of Exercise: Responses and Adaptations* (2nd edition). New York: Macmillan Publishing Company, pp: 32–37, 239–242, 260–271, 294–300, 311–321.

McArdle, W. D., F. I. Katch, and V. L. Katch (1991). *Exercise Physiology: Energy, Nutrition, and Human Performance* (3rd edition). Philadelphia: Lea & Febiger, pp: 200-211, 359–366, 452–477.

Montoye, H. J., and D. E. Lamphiear (1977). Grip and arm strength in males and females, age 10 to 69. *Research Quarterly* 8(1):109–120.

Noble, B. J. (1986). *Physiology of Exercise and Sport.* St. Louis, Missouri: Times Mirror/Mosby College Publishing, pp: 12–24, 111–122.

Powers, S. K., and E. T. Howley (1990). *Exercise Physiology: Theory and Application to Fitness and Performance.* Dubuque, Iowa: Wm. C. Brown Publishers, pp: 118–119, 156–165, 418–426, 434–444, 454.

Wilmore, J. H., and D. L. Costill (1988). *Training for Sport and Activity: The Physiological Basis of the Conditioning Process* (3rd edition). Dubuque, Iowa: Wm. C. Brown Publishers, pp. 9–17, 125–139, 372–373.

STATION 1
. . . .
Muscular Strength

Research Questions

1. Which person in your lab group has the greatest absolute strength for the bench press exercise? Which person has the greatest relative strength (strength-to-weight ratio)?

2. Describe a possible advantage and limitation for using a 1 RM to evaluate strength. Describe a possible advantage and limitation for using strength-to-weight ratios to evaluate strength.

3. Which of the above two methods do you think is the ideal way to evaluate one's improvement in muscular strength as a result of training? Defend your answer.

Data Collection

1. Use the Universal gym bench press (or comparable alternative) to determine the bench press 1 RM for each member of your lab group.

   1 RM Instructions:
   a. Assume a grip slightly wider than shoulder-width.
   b. Perform 5 to 6 submaximal repetitions to warm-up.
   c. Select a resistance (approximately 60% of body weight) and perform one repetition.
   d. Increase or decrease the weight 5 to 10 lbs until the maximum weight which can be lifted (one time) is determined.
      Note: A 1 RM lift is valid only when complete extension of the arms is realized.
   e. Rest at least one minute between repetitions. (Rotate to other lab members between repetitions to speed up the process.)
   f. Keep your feet on the floor and your back flat on the bench during the lift. Breath out (exhale) as you lift the weight.
   g. Lower the weight gently back to the start position after a given lift. Do not allow the weight to fall hard onto the weight stack.

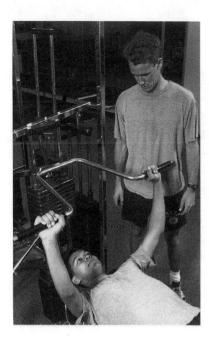

2. Compute a strength-to-weight ratio for each person in your lab group. A computation example is outlined below.

Strength-to-weight ratio = 1 RM (pounds or kg*)
Body wt (pounds or kg*)

$$\text{Strength-to-weight ratio} = \frac{1 \text{ RM (pounds or kg*)}}{\text{Body wt (pounds or kg*)}}$$

Example: 1 RM = 440 pounds

Body wt = 220 pounds

$$\text{Ratio} = \frac{440 \text{ pounds}}{220 \text{ pounds}} = \frac{220 \text{ kg}}{110 \text{ kg}} = 2.0$$

* Be sure that the unit values are the same for the both the numerator and denominator.

3. Record your results in Chart 2–1.

Name: _____ Date: _____

Muscular Strength
Assignment

STATION 1

Chart 2–1 **Strength-to-Weight Ratio** **Data Sheet**					
Name	1 RM (lbs)	1 RM (kg*)	Body Weight (lbs)	Body Weight (kg)	Ratio
1					
2					
3					
4					
5					

*Note: 1.0 kg is equivalent to 2.2 lbs.

Research Conclusions

1. Which person in your lab group has the greatest absolute strength for the bench press exercise? Which person has the greatest relative strength (strength-to-weight ratio)?

2. Describe a possible advantage and limitation for using a 1 RM to evaluate strength. Describe a possible advantage and limitation for using strength-to-weight ratios to evaluate strength.

— Machine used (in 10 pd intervals)

— Muscle Strength may vary in the individual

3. Which of the above two methods do you think is the best way to evaluate one's improvement in muscular strength as a result of training? Defend your answer.

STATION 2
Muscular Endurance

Research Questions

1. Does a stronger person have a greater, lesser, or the same absolute muscular endurance as a weaker person? Why?

2. How would you plot the relationship between muscular strength and absolute endurance (i.e., positive or negative relationship)?

3. Was the blood flow to and from the working muscle likely hampered in your subjects? Provide evidence. How might this affect the muscular endurance of your subjects?

4. Do you think a stronger person has greater, lesser, or the same relative muscular endurance as a weaker person? Justify your answer.

Data Collection

1. Determine the strongest and weakest persons in your group by performing 1 RM biceps curls with dumbbells.

   To control the lifting technique:
   a. Stand erect with your back against a wall throughout the entire lift.
   b. Start each lift with your arm fully extended.
   c. End each lift with your arm fully flexed.
   d. Record the results in Chart 2–2.

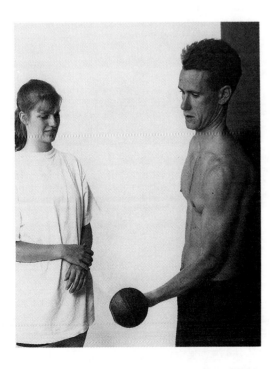

2. Select a lighter weight dumbbell of 5 to 15 lbs, and have both the strongest and weakest persons in your group perform as many repetitions as possible using a dumbbell of the same weight.

To control the experiment:
a. Implement the same control that was used when performing the initial 1 RM's.
b. Have both persons perform repetitions at the same rate.
c. Have other members of the group count each person's repetitions.
d. Record the results in Chart 2–2.
   Note: A person is considered fatigued when the individual can no longer maintain a given exercise intensity (i.e., keep up with the prescribed repetition cadence).

Muscular Endurance
Assignment

STATION 2

	1 RM (lbs)	Dumbbell Weight (lbs)	Number of Repetitions
Chart 2–2 **Muscular Endurance** Data Sheet			
Strongest Person			
Weakest Person			

Research Conclusions

1. Does a stronger person have a greater, lesser, or the same absolute muscular endurance as a weaker person? Why?

   Jeremy – 1RM = 68 pds # of reps = 120   Strongest greater
   Julie – 1RM = 17 pds # of reps = 20   ME than weakest

   but LeAnn – 1RM = 22 pds # of reps = 16 less
   + Michelle – 1RM = 22 pds # of reps = 20 same   Normally,
   has stronger person greater ME

2. How would you plot the relationship between muscular strength and absolute endurance (i.e., positive or negative relationship)?

3. Was the blood flow to and from the working muscle likely hampered in your subjects? Provide evidence. How might this affect the muscular endurance of your subjects?

4. Based on your findings, do you think a stronger person has greater, lesser, or the same relative muscular endurance as a weaker person? Justify your answer.

STATION 3

. . . .
Assessment Of Muscular Fitness

Part I

Research Questions

1. If a national mailing/parcel service required a minimum strength score of 85 points in order for an individual to be considered for employment, would the average male and female student enrolled in this laboratory class satisfy this criteria? Provide results.

2. Does this appear to be an acceptable test for a parcel service to use for screening job applicants? Justify your answer.

Data Collection

1. Perform the strength test outlined below. Wear lightweight and nonrestrictive clothing. Be sure to avoid strenuous exercise for several hours before the test.

2. Determine the recommended exercise weight for each lift by computing the appropriate percentage of your total body weight. Record your exercise weights in Chart 2–3.

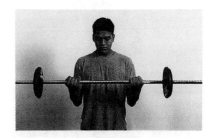

Computation example for the arm curl exercise:

Male: Body Weight(lbs) × % Body Weight = Exercise Weight

156 lbs × 35% (or 0.35) = 54.6 or 55 lbs.

Female: Body Weight(lbs) × % Body Weight = Exercise Weight

123 lbs × 18% (or 0.18) = 22.14 or 22 lbs.

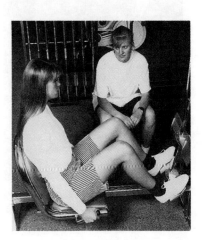

3. Perform each exercise in the order shown in Chart 2–3. Complete as many repetitions as possible. Record the number of repetitions performed for each exercise in Chart 2–3.

4. Record your points and fitness category for each exercise based on scores outlined in Table 2–1. (Example: If a female performed 14 repetitions for the arm-curl exercise, a score of 13 points would be earned. This score would be considered in the Very Good category.)

5. Add up your total points to determine your overall test results. Based on Table 2–2 determine your overall norm rating.

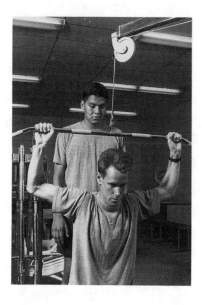

6. Record your total points as well as the total points of each member of your lab in the class summary Chart 2–4. Compute the class total and class average. Use the norm chart (Table 2–2) to determine the average class rating.

Table 2–1
Muscular Fitness Scoring Table

Fitness Category	Points	Male	Female	Male	Female
		ARM CURL		BENCH PRESS	
Very Poor	5	≤ 2	≤ 2	0	0
Poor	7	3–4	3–5	1–2	1
Fair	9	5–7	6–7	3–6	2–4
Good	11	8–9	8–11	7–10	5–9
Very Good	13	10–14	12–15	11–15	10–15
Excellent	15	15–20	16–20	16–20	16–20
Superior	17	21+	21+	21+	21+
		LAT PULLDOWN		LEG EXTENSION	
Very Poor	5	0–3	0–2	0–3	0–1
Poor	7	4–5	3–5	4–6	2–4
Fair	9	6–8	6–8	7–9	5–7
Good	11	9–10	9–10	10–12	8–9
Very Good	13	11–15	11–15	13–14	10–12
Excellent	15	16–24	16–24	15–19	13–19
Superior	17	25+	25+	20+	20+
		LEG CURL		Abd CURL UP	
Very Poor	5	0–1	0	0–22	0–14
Poor	7	2–3	1–2	23–27	15–19
Fair	9	4–7	3–4	28–32	20–24
Good	11	8–10	5–6	33–36	25–29
Very Good	13	11–14	7–9	37–40	30–33
Excellent	15	15–19	10–16	41–44	34–38
Superior	17	20+	17+	45+	39+

Source: Adapted from Hoeger (1991).

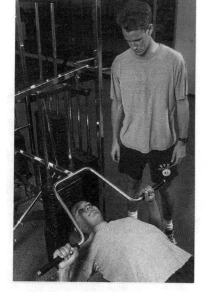

Table 2–2
Strength Fitness Norm Chart

Category	Total Points
Poor	< 54
Fair	54–65
Good	66–77
Very Good	78–89
Excellent	> 89

*Adapted from Hoeger (1989).

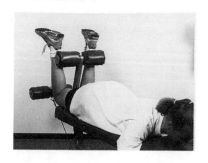

Name: _____ Date: _____

Assessment of Muscular Fitness
Assignment

STATION 3
Part I

Chart 2–3 **Muscular Strength and Endurance Test** **Individual Data Sheet**						
Body Weight: _____ lbs; _____ kg						
Body Height: _____ inches; _____ cm						
Age: _____ Gender: _____						
Exercise	*Male % BW*	*Female %BW*	*Exercise Wt (lbs)*	*Reps*	*Points*	*Fitness Category*
Two-Arm Biceps Curl	35	18				
Leg Extension	65	50				
Lat Pulldown	70	45				
1-Minute Timed Sit-Up						
Bench Press	75	45				
Leg Curl	32	25				
Total Points and Overall Rating:						

Source: Adapted from Hoeger (1989).

Chart 2–4
Muscular Strength and Endurance
Class Data Sheet

Male		Female	
Subject	Strength Score	Subject	Strength Score
1		1	
2		2	
3		3	
4		4	
5		5	
6		6	
7		7	
8		8	
9		9	
10		10	
11		11	
12		12	
13		13	
14		14	
15		15	
Total		Total	
Average		Average	
Rating		Rating	

Research Conclusions

1. If a national mailing/parcel service required a minimum strength score of 85 points in order for an individual to be considered for employment, would the average male and female student enrolled in this laboratory class satisfy this criterion? What percentage of the class passed this criterion score of 85 points? Do these results appear realistic for the students in your class?

2. Does this appear to be an acceptable test for a parcel service to use for screening job applicants? Justify your answer.

STATION 3

∙ ∙

Assessment Of Muscular Fitness

Part II

Research Questions

1. Could a national parcel service use a hand-grip test to evaluate an applicant's strength instead of the strength test used in Part I of Station 3? Explain the various pros and cons of making such a change.

2. Are you classified in a different category for the grip test than the other strength test? Why might you be classified in the same or different category? Explain.

3. Do you think the parcel service should consider any other components of physical fitness when evaluating job applicants? If so, which components should they consider and why?

Data Collection

Perform the grip test according to the following test protocol:

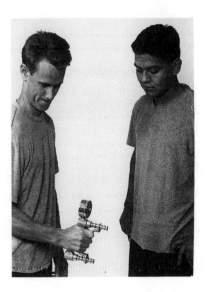

1. Assume a standing position with your head erect, facing straight forward.
2. Adjust the grip dynamometer so that the middle finger's second phalanx opposes the gripping device at a 90° angle.
3. Set your forearm at a 45° angle and rotate the forearm slightly outward.
4. Squeeze the hand-grip dynamometer quickly and maximally, taking no more than a few seconds to perform each trial. Do not move from your initial body position.
5. Perform two or three trials alternately with each hand. Rest approximately 20 to 60 seconds between each trial.
6. After each trial record your results in Chart 2–5. Based on Table 2–3 determine your normative rating.

Table 2–3
Hand Grip Norm Chart for Ages 20–29
(Sum of right and left hand in kg)

Fitness Category	Male	Female
Poor	< 68	< 35
Fair	68–86	35–46
Average	87–104	47–58
Good	105–122	59–70
Excellent	> 122	> 71

Source: Adapted from the Canadian Public Health Association Project (1977).

Assessment of Muscular Fitness
Assignment

STATION 3
Part II

Chart 2–5				
Individual Grip Test Data Sheet				
Right Hand		Left Hand		
Trial #	Score (kg)	Trial #	Score (kg)	Sum of both hands (kg)
1	30	1	28	58
2	28.5	2	27.5	56
3	30	3	28.5	58.5
Fitness Rating:				

Research Conclusions

1. Could a national parcel service use a hand-grip test to evaluate an applicant's strength instead of the strength test used in Part I of Station 3? Explain the various pros and cons of making such a change.

2. Are you classified in a different category for the grip test than the other strength test? Why might you be classified in the same or different category? Explain.

3. Do you think this parcel service should consider any other components of physical fitness when evaluating job applicants? If so, which components should they consider and why?

. . . .
Lab 2 Summary

Describe several ways the information learned in this lab can be applied to your chosen field of interest and/or your personal life. Be specific and provide practical examples.

3

Flexibility
. . . .
Pre-Laboratory Assignment

1. If a swimmer questioned the importance of a flexibility training program, describe two things you could say to impress upon her the need for such a program.

2. Outline at least three basic principles that should be followed when stretching.

3. Name a sport or activity that requires a significant amount of flexibility. Describe a stretching exercise that would increase the joint range of motion for an important movement used in this sport.

4. ☐ Check the box if you have read each research question for this lab and are familiar with the data collection procedures regarding each research question.

3

Flexibility

PURPOSE
The purpose of this lab is to allow you to measure and evaluate flexibility.

STUDENT LEARNING OBJECTIVES
1. Be able to administer the traditional and modified sit-and-reach tests and understand how to evaluate these tests.
2. Be able to justify the importance of flexibility fitness.

NECESSARY EQUIPMENT
Sit-and-reach board
Meterstick
Leighton flexometer or goniometer

All five components of physical fitness are important, yet joint range of motion or flexibility is a component often overlooked. Flexibility is the ability to move a specific body part through a prescribed joint range of motion, and is dependent on the looseness or suppleness of the muscles, tendons, and ligaments that surround a given joint. The integrity of the joint capsule itself can also affect flexibility. Limited flexibility is usually the result of muscles and tendons that are too tight; however, excess fat can also be a contributing factor.

Flexibility training is an important part of any exercise program because a satisfactory level of flexibility can enhance one's ability to carry out many daily activities. Increased flexibility also appears to improve posture, reduce the likelihood of low-back problems, enhance athletic performance, and decrease the risk of recreational and sports-related injuries.

Proper stretching techniques are easy to learn. However, there are a few rules to keep in mind.

1. Warm-up the muscles you wish to stretch by performing whole-body activities (i.e., cycling, jogging) or simple calisthenics immediately before you stretch. Warm-up for at least 3 minutes.
2. Perform a slow, easy stretch. Extend to a point where you feel only mild tension and then relax as you hold the stretch. Do not bounce.
3. Hold each stretch for 10 to 30 seconds and practice good technique.
4. Relax and maintain a normal breathing pattern as you hold your stretch.

SELECTED REFERENCES
American College of Sports Medicine (1991). *Guidelines of Exercise Testing and Prescription* (4th edition). Philadelphia: Lea & Febiger, pp: 48–54.

Anderson, B. (1980). *Stretching*. Bolinas, California: Shelter Publications.

Canadian Public Health Assocation Project (1977). Fitness and Amateur Sport, Canada.

Corbin, C. (1984). Flexibility. *Clinical Sports Medicine* 3:101–117.

Fisher, A. G., and C. R. Jensen (1990). *Scientific Basis of Athletic Conditioning* (3rd edition). Philadelphia: Lea & Febiger, pp: 265–266.

Fox, E. L., R. W. Bowers, and M. L. Foss (1988). *The Physiological Basis of Physical Education and Athletics* (4th edition). Philadelphia: Saunders College Publishing, pp: 188–194.

Harris, M.L. (1969). A factor analytic study of flexibility. *Research Quarterly* 49: 62–70.

Heyward, V. H. (1991). *Advanced Fitness Assessment and Exercise Prescription*. Champaign, Illinois: Human Kinetic Books, pp: 215–229.

Hoeger, W.W.K. (1991). *Principles and Labs for Physical Fitness and Wellness*. Englewood, Colorado: Morton Publishing.

Hoeger, W. W. K. (1989). *Lifetime Physical Fitness and Wellness: A Personalized Program*. Englewood, Colorado: Morton Publishing Company, pp: 81–99.

Lamb, D. R. (1984). *Physiology of Exercise: Responses and Adaptations* (2nd edition). New York: Macmillan Publishing Company, pp: 371–373.

Powers, S. K., and E. T. Howley (1990). *Exercise Physiology: Theory and Application to Fitness and Performance*. Dubuque, Iowa: Wm. C. Brown Publishers, pp: 456–457.

Wilmore, J. H., and D. L. Costill (1988). *Training for Sport and Activity: The Physiological Basis of the Conditioning Process* (3rd edition). Dubuque, Iowa: Wm. C. Brown Publishers, pp: 373–375.

STATION 1

· · · · · · · · · · · · · · · · · · · ·

Flexibility Assessment

Research Questions

1. Is there a difference in your flexibility fitness rating when using the traditional versus the modified sit-and-reach tests? Describe your results.

2. Is the modified sit-and-reach test a more valid test of flexibility than the traditional sit-and-reach test? Defend your answer.

3. Outline three sources of error that may have biased your results.

Data Collection

Wearing comfortable, non-restricting clothing, perform the traditional and modified sit-and-reach tests according to the following instructions. Note that both tests estimate the flexibility of the lower back, hip extensor, and knee flexor muscles.

Traditional Sit-and-Reach Test

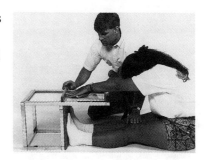

1. Perform simple calisthenics and static stretching for at least 3 minutes to warm-up your low back and legs prior to the test.
2. Remove your shoes and assume a sitting position on the floor. Extend your legs straight in front of you and press your feet against the measurement apparatus.
3. Place one hand on top of the other and reach forward as far as possible. Exhale as you stretch forward.
4. Perform 3 trials keeping the backs of your legs firmly on the floor while stretching. Do not bounce; stretch slow and easy.
5. Have your partner note the farthest point reached on the third trial. Record your results in Chart 3–1. Note that the zero centimeter mark is where the feet contact the box. Adjust the normative values (see Table 3–1) accordingly if your measurement box utilizes different measurement units.
6. Based on the norms in Table 3–1 determine your flexibility rating for the traditional sit-and-reach test. Record your results in Chart 3–1.

Table 3–1
Flexibility Norm Chart for Sit-and-Reach Tests

Rating	Traditional* (cm)		Modified† (cm)	
	Males	Females	Males	Females
Poor	< 14.0	< 30.0	< 29.5	< 32.0
Fair	14.0–24.0	30.0–33.0	29.5–34.0	32.0–36.5
Average	24.1–35.0	33.1–37.0	34.1–38.0	36.6–40.0
Good	35.1–45.0	37.1–41.0	38.1–43.0	40.1–42.0
Excellent	> 45.0	> 41.0	> 43.0	> 42.0

*Source: Adapted from Canadian Public Health Association Project (1977); for ages 20–29; footline set at 25 centimeters.

†Source: Adapted from Hoeger (1991), for ages 19–35 yr.

Modified Sit-and-Reach Test

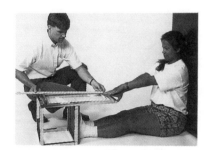

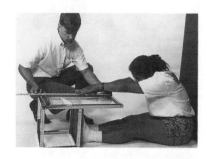

1. Perform simple calisthenics and static stretching for at least 3 minutes to warm-up your low back and legs prior to the test.
2. Remove your shoes and assume a sitting position on the floor. Extend your legs straight in front of you and press your feet against the measurement box. Keep your legs straight.
3. Establish your starting position as follows: Position your back against a wall. Place one hand on top of the other and reach forward as far as possible without letting your head and back break contact with the wall. You may round your shoulders as much as possible, but neither your head nor back should come off the wall. Have your partner position a meterstick on the top of the box so that the end of the meterstick touches your fingers and is pointed directly (straight) away from you. This becomes the starting position (0 centimeters) for the test. The meterstick must be held firmly in place throughout the remainder of the test.
4. From this starting position perform three trials. Exhale as you stretch forward keeping the backs of your legs firmly on the floor. Do not bounce; stretch slowly and easily.
5. Have your partner note the farthest point reached along the meterstick on the third trial. Record your score to the nearest centimeter in Chart 3–1.

Name: _____ Date: _____

Flexibility Assessment
Assignment

STATION 1

Chart 3–1	
Individual Flexibility Results	
Traditional sit-and-reach score (cm):	
Modified sit-and-reach score (cm):	

Research Conclusions

1. Is there a difference in your sit-and-reach score when using the traditional versus modified method? Discuss differences.

2. Is the modified sit-and-reach test a more valid test of flexibility than the traditional sit-and-reach test? Defend your answer.

3. Outline three sources of error that may have biased your results.

FLEXIBILITY

STATION 2
. . . .
Flexibility Training

Research Questions

1. Does a single flexibility training session increase the average flexibility score in your class by at least 10%? Describe and discuss results.

2. Describe at least two ways flexibility training can increase joint range of motion. (Provide physiologically sound principles).

3. Explain how increased flexibility of the low back may help you reduce your risk of low-back problems. Explain how the other four components of health-related physical fitness may help to reduce low-back problems.

Data Collection

1. Perform the modified sit-and-reach test prior to a session of flexibility training. Record your pre-test score on the class data sheet (Chart 3–2).
2. Your instructor will lead your lab class in various stretching exercises designed to improve your sit-and-reach score.
3. Warm-up properly. Perform slow, comfortable stretches. Hold your stretch for 10–30 seconds. Maintain a normal breathing pattern.
4. Your flexibility training session should be thorough. Plan to take at least 15–20 minutes completing your session. Be sure that you continue stretching up to the time you are evaluated.
5. Perform the modified sit-and-reach test after your flexibility training session. Record your post-test score on the class data sheet (Chart 3–2).
6. Calculate the percent change between the class's first and second sit-and-reach score.

Alternative Activity

Use a goniometer or Leighton flexometer to measure a single joint movement; i.e., trunk flexion. (Your instructor will demonstrate how to use this equipment.) Perform a session of flexibility training as discussed above. Record class pre- and post-training flexibility scores in Chart 3–2. Compute percent change scores and complete the research conclusions.

Name:_____   Date: _____

Flexibility Assessment

STATION 2

	Chart 3–2		
	Class Data Sheet		
	Flexibility Training		
Subject	Pre-Test	Post-Test	% Change*
1			
2			
3			
4			
5			
6			
7			
8			
9			
10			
11			
12			
13			
14			
15			
16			
17			
18			
19			
20			
Total			
Average			

*Note: % Change $= \dfrac{\text{Post-Test} - \text{Pre-Test}}{\text{Pre-Test}} \times 100$

Research Conclusions

1. Does a single flexibility training session increase the average flexibility score in your class by at least 10%? Describe and discuss results.

2. Describe at least two ways flexibility training can increase joint range of motion. (Provide physiologically sound principles.)

3. Explain how increased flexibility of the low back may help you reduce your risk of low-back problems. Explain how the other four components of health-related physical fitness may help to reduce low back problems.

Name: _____   Date: _____

Lab 3 Summary

Describe several ways the information learned in this lab can be applied in your chosen field of interest and/or your personal life. Be specific and provide practical examples.

Name: _____   Date: _____

4

Heart Rate
and Blood Pressure
. . . .
Pre-Laboratory Assignment

1. Describe four ways to increase the accuracy and consistency of resting heart rate measurements.

2. If you counted 15 beats in a 10-second period of time, what would be the heart rate? Show work.

3. Describe how the timed heart rate method is different from the 30-beat heart rate method.

4. Briefly outline the procedure for measuring resting blood pressure.

5. How does the miscounting of 1 beat affect the beats-per-minute computation for the 6-, 10-, 15-, and 30-second timed heart rate method? Show your work.

6. ❑ Check the box if you have read each research question and are familiar with the data collection procedures regarding each research question.

4

Heart Rate and Blood Pressure

HEART RATE

The rate of the cardiac cycle (heart rate) provides important insight into what is happening in the body at rest and during exercise. A low resting heart rate (HR) (bradycardia–HR < 60 bpm) may indicate a well-conditioned heart that is able to pump large amounts of blood with each beat. Conversely, a high resting heart rate (tachycardia–HR > 100 bpm) may be indicative of a poorly-conditioned heart. Resting HR is affected by several factors including body position, diet, consumption of drugs, alcohol, or caffeine, and fatigue.

Individuals who are involved in a rigorous regimen of exercise are commonly advised to measure resting HR immediately upon waking in the morning since high resting HRs (> 5 bpm above normal) often suggest overtraining. The advice given to an athlete with an abnormally high resting HR would be to cut back on training until normal resting HRs were realized. Such knowledge is valuable as athletes seek to reach levels of peak performance and avoid over-use injuries.

Generally, males have lower resting HR values than females. For example, males often demonstrate resting HRs between 60–70 bpm and females between 70–80 bpm. A few reasons for this difference is that females, on average, pump less blood per beat (lower stroke volume), transport less oxygen per volume of blood (because of less hemoglobin), and have a lower total blood volume than do males. Overall, the average population resting HR is approximately 72 bpm.

In order to measure true resting heart rate it is important to control several factors:

1. Drug and medication consumption. Many drugs (i.e., caffeine, tobacco, alcohol, prescription medication) directly affect HR. Thus it is recommended

to abstain from consuming these chemicals for at least 12 hours before measuring resting HR.

2. Body position. Skeletal muscle activity is a strong stimulant for increased HR. A resting, supine body position is best during testing.

3. Dietary status. It takes energy to digest food and HRs increase in order to deliver needed blood to metabolically active tissues (i.e., gut).

4. Environmental factors. Noise, temperature extremes, and pollution can increase stress. The body's attempt to overcome stress requires an expenditure of energy which can increase resting HR. Accordingly, it is best to minimize environmental extremes as much as possible when measuring resting HR.

During exercise a person's HR indirectly indicates exercise intensity or exertion levels. Since the heart plays a pivotal role in supplying oxygen and nutrients (i.e., glucose, fats, etc.) and removing wastes (i.e., carbon dioxide, metabolic acids, etc.), the rate of the cardiac cycle is a valid indicator of the demands required of the body. Exercise HR is commonly used to help an individual utilize a specific energy system (i.e., aerobic, anaerobic) and/or condition specific systems of the body (i.e., cardiovascular, respiratory, etc.).

Several types of equipment and methods are used to measure HR.

1. **Electrocardiogram (ECG)** An important medical instrument used in the diagnosis of cardiovascular disease. In exercise science the ECG is generally used to screen for potential cardiovascular abnormalities during and/or following exercise. The ECG is also used to monitor heart rate and cardiac function at rest and during exercise.

2. **Telemetry equipment** (heart rate monitors) Telemetry involves the transmission of a signal from an adjustable chest harness to an electronic receiver that can be hand held or attached to the wrist. The receiver converts the signal from the chest harness into a quantified HR measurement. Recent research has indicated that telemetry devices can accurately measure both resting and exercise HR.

3. **Palpation** Feeling a pulse or vibration with the fingers or hand is termed palpation. The pulse, generated by the pulsatile pumping of blood in the arteries, is most easily felt over the radial or carotid arteries. When taking a pulse to measure

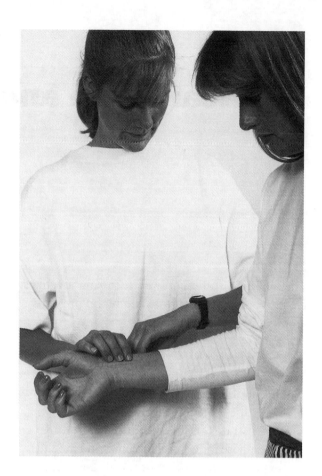

HR, remember to press lightly with the fingers to avoid occluding (obstructing) the blood flow.

An apical beat (vibration pulse) is generated by the left ventricle hitting the chest wall near the left fifth rib. The apical beat can be quite prominent in lean individuals immediately following exercise. To palpate an apical beat, position the entire hand over the left side of the chest (as in the Pledge of Allegiance).

4. **Stethoscope** Auscultatory (by ear) HRs are more accurate than palpation methods. In fact, a stethoscope is nearly as accurate in measuring HR as electrocardiography (ECG) equipment. The basic purpose of the stethoscope is to amplify and direct sound waves, thus bringing the ear of the listener closer to the source of the sound.

To use a stethoscope:

a. Insert the ear tips of the stethoscope directly down each ear canal so that the ear tips of the stethoscope point forward. If you fail to position the ear tips properly it will be difficult to hear the heart beat.

b. Gently tap the diaphragm of the stethoscope to

be sure you can pick up sound through the stethoscope.

c. Position the stethoscope just below the left breast and/or pectoralis major muscle. The diaphragm of the stethoscope should be held firmly against the skin. Placing the stethoscope over clothing increases the chances of hearing interfering sounds from external sources.

Auscultating heart beats at rest with a stethoscope is often more difficult than during exercise since the heart sounds are less pronounced. However, with practice one can become skilled at measuring resting HR with a stethoscope.

Within the research and clinical setting, ECG or telemetric techniques are the preferred methods for measuring HR. In a more practical setting, however, it is important to know how to measure HR using both a stethoscope and palpation. Outlined below is a brief explanation of two methods used to measure HR.

The *Timed Heart Rate Method* simply requires counting the number of pulses in a specific amount of time. Usually pulse counts are taken for 6, 10, or 15 seconds. If the pulse is taken for 6 seconds, the pulse count is multiplied by 10; if the pulse is taken for 10 seconds, the pulse count is multiplied by 6; and if the pulse is taken for 15 seconds, the pulse count is multiplied by 4. An alternative way to compute the HR is to use the formula outlined below:

For example:

$$\text{HR (bpm)} = \frac{\text{beats counted}}{\text{time (sec)}} \times \frac{60 \text{ seconds}}{1 \text{ minute}}$$

$$90 \text{ bpm} = \frac{15 \text{ beats}}{10 \text{ sec}} \times \frac{60 \text{ seconds}}{1 \text{ minute}}$$

The *30-Beat Heart Rate Method* requires measuring the amount of time for 30 heart beats to occur. A formula and computation example for this method are below:

$$\text{HR (bpm)} = \frac{30 \text{ beats}}{\text{time (sec)}} \times \frac{60 \text{ seconds}}{1 \text{ minute}}$$

$$90 \text{ bpm} = \frac{30 \text{ beats}}{20 \text{ sec}} \times \frac{60 \text{ seconds}}{1 \text{ minute}}$$

Note: For this method, count the first beat as "zero" and simultaneously begin your stop watch. A conversion chart for this method is outlined in Table 4–1.

The measurement of HR *during* weight-bearing

Table 4–1
Conversion Chart for 30-Beat Heart Rate Method*

Time for 30 Beats (sec)	Heart Rate (bpm)	Time for 30 Beats (sec)	Heart Rate (bpm)
30.0	60	19.0	95
29.5	61	18.5	97
29.0	62	18.0	100
28.5	63	17.5	103
28.0	64	17.0	106
27.5	65	16.5	109
27.0	67	16.0	113
26.5	68	15.5	116
26.0	69	15.0	120
25.5	71	14.5	124
25.0	72	14.0	129
24.5	73	13.5	133
24.0	75	13.0	138
23.5	77	12.5	144
23.0	78	12.0	150
22.5	80	11.5	157
22.0	82	11.0	164
21.5	84	10.5	171
21.0	86	10.0	180
20.5	88	9.5	189
20.0	90	9.0	200
19.5	92	8.5	212

*HRs are rounded to nearest whole number.

exercise (i.e., walking, running, cycling) is best performed with either ECG or telemetry equipment. If such equipment is unavailable, exercise HR can be estimated after exercise by using either the palpation or auscultation method. However, because the HR can drop rapidly following exercise, begin timing pulse counts as quickly as possible!

BLOOD PRESSURE

Blood pressure is defined as an outward force that distends blood vessel walls. The magnitude of blood pressure depends primarily on the volume of blood (blood flow) and the size of the vessel (vascular resistance). The unit for expressing blood pressure is typically millimeters of mercury (mm Hg).

Blood pressure, from a health and fitness standpoint, is most commonly measured within the arteries. The standard site of blood pressure determination is the brachial artery. Selecting the brachial artery as the standard site of measurement is due to convenience, accessibility, and its position at heart level.

In the laboratory setting, blood pressure is determined indirectly by listening to Korotkoff sounds, which are sounds made from vibrations along the vascular walls. The equipment needed to detect these sounds are a stethoscope and cuff manometer (sphygmomanometer). The manometer (gauge) used to quantify blood pressure can be either aneroid or mercury.

Korotkoff sounds are only present when the vascular wall is deformed in some way. If the vessel wall is round and symmetrical, no vibration sounds can be detected. The blood pressure cuff is used to change the shape of the vessel wall and facilitate Korotkoff sounds. By inflating the air bladder in the cuff, the walls of the brachial artery become compressed. As blood attempts to flow past the compressed area, turbulent blood flow causes the arterial wall to vibrate and sounds are detected with the stethoscope. There are five different Korotkoff sounds or phases that are used to define blood pressure. However, we will concern ourselves primarily with the first, fourth, and fifth phases (Figure 4–1).

Systolic blood pressure (SBP), the pressure exerted against the brachial artery as the heart muscle contracts, is indicated by the first Korotkoff sound. The first step in measuring blood pressure is inflating the cuff so that the blood flow through the brachial artery is completely occluded. At this point no vibration sounds can be heard. As the air bladder of the cuff is slowly deflated, the blood pressure within the vessel overcomes the cuff pressure and a bolus of blood flows through the brachial artery. This initial blood flow produces a Korotkoff sound (Phase 1) and indirectly represents the peak blood pressure or systolic blood pressure.

Diastolic blood pressure (DBP), the pressure exerted against the brachial artery when the heart is relaxed, is indicated by the fourth and fifth Korotkoff sounds. As the cuff pressure is continuously released, blood pressure within the vessel increases and eventually exceeds the cuff pressure. At this point the blood pressure distends the vessel wall back to its

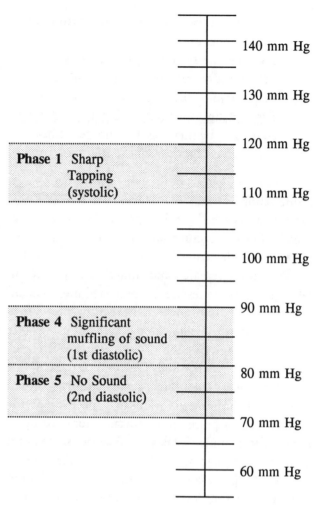

Figure 4–1. Blood pressure vs. Korotokoff sounds. Major phases of the Korotkoff sounds when systolic pressure (Phase 1) is 120 mm Hg, and diastolic pressures (Phase 4 and 5) are 90 and 80 mm Hg, respectively.

original shape and the Korotkoff sounds will fade (Phase 4) then disappear (Phase 5). (See Figure 4–1.)

Note: For adults with normal blood pressure, the fifth Korotkoff sound (pressure at which the Korotkoff sounds disappear) is used to indicate diastolic blood pressure. However, for children and adults who have Korotkoff sounds below 40 mm Hg, the fourth Korotkoff phase is used. Blood pressure is recorded as SBP over DBP.

An effort should be made to minimize the following sources of measurement error when taking blood pressure:

- Auditory acuity of test administrator
- Background noise
- Experience of test administrator
- Improper cuff width or length

- Improper stethoscope placement and pressure
- Inaccurate sphygmomanometer
- Rate of inflation or deflation of the cuff pressure
- Reaction time of the test administrator*

*Source: Morehouse (1972)

Blood pressure is measured at rest (in the standing and supine positions) and during exercise. At rest, blood pressure is used to screen for hyper- or hypotension. In addition, resting blood pressure is used to evaluate the influence medications may have on the cardiovascular system.

Normal resting blood pressure is considered to be 120/80 (numerator = systolic blood pressure; denominator = diastolic blood pressure). Some individuals have higher than normal blood pressure levels, which result in the condition known as hypertension. The National Heart and Blood Institute has classified normal and hypertensive levels of blood pressure as follows:

Resting Diastolic Blood Pressure

Normal:	< 90 mm Hg
Mild hypertension:	90–104 mm Hg
Moderate hypertension:	105–114 mm Hg
Severe hypertension:	> 114 mm Hg

Resting Systolic Blood Pressure

Normal:	< 140 mm Hg
Borderline hypertension:	140–159 mm Hg
Isolated hypertension:	> 159 mm Hg

During exercise, measuring blood pressure is routinely used to determine the normality of blood pressure responses and assess the influence medications have on functional capacity. As a result of exercise, systolic blood pressure is expected to rise due to an increase in cardiac output. Diastolic blood pressure, on the other hand, is expected to remain equivalent to resting levels or decrease during exercise due to increased vasodilation and opening of capillary beds. Typical exercise blood pressure values are:

Systolic:	150 to 200 mm Hg
Diastolic:	Remain the same as at resting or may slightly decrease during exercise.

Individuals who have cardiovascular disease may have abnormal blood pressure responses to exercise. Exercise or exercise testing is usually terminated if blood pressure responses are abnormal. Contraindicated* exercise blood pressure responses include:

- A drop in systolic blood pressure of 20 mm Hg or more or an increase in systolic blood pressure to 250 mm Hg or more.
- A rise in diastolic blood pressure to 120 mm Hg or more.

* Contraindications: Unfavorable indications or signs that provide grounds for stopping an exercise test.

SELECTED REFERENCES

Adams, G. M. *Exercise Physiology Lab Manual* (1990). Dubuque, Iowa: Wm. C. Brown Publishers, pp: 117–131.

American College of Sports Medicine. (1991). *Guidelines of Exercise Testing and Prescription* (4th edition). Philadelphia: Lea & Febiger, pp: 19–22, 69, 72.

American Heart Association: Recommendation for Human Blood Pressure Determination by Sphygmomanometers, Dallas, 1980.

DeVries, H. A. (1986). *Physiology of Exercise: For Physical Education and Athletics* (4th edition). Dubuque, Iowa: Wm. C. Brown Publishers, pp: 120–124, 139–140.

Fisher, A. G., and C. R. Jensen (1990). *Scientific Basis of Athletic Conditioning* (3rd edition). Philadelphia: Lea & Febiger, pp: 86–88, 95–98.

Heyward, V. H. (1991). *Advanced Fitness Assessment and Exercise Prescription*. Champaign, Illinois: Human Kinetic, pp: 18–22.

Howley, E. T., and D. B. Frank (1992). *Health Fitness Instructor's Handbook* (2nd edition). Champaign, Illinois: Human Kinetics, pp: 42–46, 164–165.

Kaufman, F. L., R. L. Hughson, and J. P. Schman (1987). Effect of exercise on recovery blood pressure in normotensive and hypertensive subjects. *Medicine and Science in Sports and Exercise* 19(1):17–20.

King, G.E. (1969). Taking the blood pressure. *Journal of the American Medical Assn* 209(12):1902–1904.

Lamb, D. R. (1984). *Physiology of Exercise: Responses and Adaptations* (2nd edition). New York: Macmillan Publishing Company, pp: 139–143, 153.

McArdle, W. D., L. Zwiren, and J. R. Magel (1969). Validity of post-exercise heart rate as a means of estimating heart rate during work of varying intensities. *Research Quarterly* 40:523–529.

McArdle, W. D., F. I. Katch, and V. L. Katch (1991). *Exercise Physiology: Energy, Nutrition, and Human Performance* (3rd edition). Philadelphia: Lea & Febiger, pp: 171, 296–297.

Morehouse, L. E. (1972). *Laboratory Manual for Physiology of Exercise*. St. Louis: Mosby.

Pollock, M. J., J. Broida, and Z. Kendrick (1972). Validity of the palpation technique of heart rate determination and its estimation of training heart rate. *Research Quarterly* 43:77–81.

Pollock, M. L. and J. H. Wilmore (1990). Exercise in Health and

Disease: Evaluation and Prescription and Rehabilitation (2nd Edition). Philadelphia: W. B. Saunders Company.Porcari, J.P., M. Robarge, and R. Veldhuis (1993). Counting heart rate right. *Fitness Managment* 9(9):44.

Powers, S. K., and E. T. Howley (1990). *Exercise Physiology: Theory and Application to Fitness and Performance.* Dubuque, Iowa: Wm. C. Brown Publishers, pp: 311–312.

Wilmore, J. H., and D. L. Costill (1988). *Training for Sport and Activity: The Physiological Basis of the Conditioning Process* (3rd edition). Dubuque, Iowa: Wm. C. Brown Publishers, pp: 72–74, 77, 158–161.

STATION 1
Measurement of Heart Rate

Research Questions

1. Which method of HR palpation measurement (Chart 4–1) should provide the most accurate resting HR results? Why?

2. How far is your resting heart rate from bradycardia and tachycardia? Does it appear that your resting heart rate is normal for your gender? Describe populations likely to have bradycardia and tachycardia.

3. What is the average difference in HR measurement between the two different administrators (Chart 4–2)? Describe at least two reasons for differences between administrators.

4. Which method of HR palpation measurement (Chart 4–3) should be used to provide the most accurate reflection of exercise HR? Why? If an electronic HR monitor was used, how do your post-exercise palpation results compare with the monitors?

Data Collection

Resting Heart Rate
1. Form groups of three and rest for about 5 minutes.
2. Have a group member measure your resting HR. Utilize each method outlined in Chart 4–1 and record the results.
3. Have two group members (administrators) measure the third member's (subject) resting HR. (Each administrator should hold one of the subject's arms and palpate the radial pulse.) Utilize each method outlined in Chart 4–2. Be sure that both administrators are unaware of each other's results. Record the results in Chart 4–2.

Exercise Heart Rate (Class Demonstration)
1. A test administrator will measure post-exercise HR by each method outlined in Chart 4–3. The subject (volunteer) should cycle at a self-

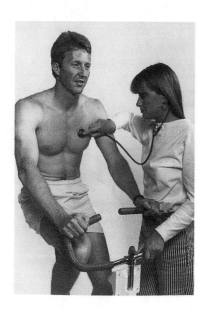

Exercise Heart Rate (Class Demonstration)

1. A test administrator will measure post-exercise HR by each method outlined in Chart 4–3. The subject (volunteer) should cycle at a self-selected moderate-exercise intensity for 2 to 3 minutes before each HR assessment.

   If a HR monitor is available, place a drop of water on the chest strap heart rate sensors and secure around the chest (against the skin, just below the sternum) of the subject. During exercise, when the HR has reached steady-state, record HR via the electronic monitor wrist-watch receiver. Keep the HR monitor results hidden from the administrator until after the experiment. Note that a single-lead ECG can be used when a HR monitor is not available.

2. Record the results in Chart 4–3.

Measurement of Heart Rate
Assignment

STATION 1

Chart 4–1 Resting Heart Rate Data Sheet		
Method	Pulse Count	Heart Rate (bpm)
30-beat HR	14 sec	
6-second timed HR	7	70
10-second timed HR	13	78
20-second timed HR	22	66
30-second timed HR	26	52
1-minute timed HR	74	74

Chart 4–2 Resting Heart Rate Data Sheet			
Administrator #1: _____ #2: _____			
	Heart Rate (bpm)		
Method	Admin #1	Admin #2	Difference
30-beat HR			
6-second timed HR			
10-second timed HR			
20-second timed HR			
30-second timed HR			
1-minute timed HR			
Average difference:			

		Chart 4–3		
	Post-Exercise Heart Rate Data Sheet			
Method	Data	Heart Rate (bpm)	Electronic Monitor* (bpm)	
10-second timed HR	Beats			
30-second timed HR	Beats			
30-beat HR	Seconds			

Note:*Heart rate should be recorded via the electronic monitor during exercise when the heart rate has reached steady-state.

Research Conclusions

1. Which method of HR palpation measurement (Chart 4–1) should provide the most accurate resting HR results? Why?

2. How far is your resting heart rate away from bradycardia and tachycardia? Does it appear that your resting heart rate is normal for your gender? Describe populations likely to have bradycardia and tachycardia.

3. What is the average difference in HR measurement between the two different administrators (Chart 4–2)? Describe at least two reasons for differences between administrators.

4. Which method of HR palpation measurement (Chart 4–3) should be used to provide the most accurate reflection of exercise HR? Why? If an electronic HR monitor was used, how do your post-exercise palpatation results compare with the monitors?

STATION 2

Measurement Of Blood Pressure

Research Questions

1. Is the average resting blood pressure in your laboratory class equal to the population average of 120/80 mm Hg? Describe at least two reasons why the lab average may be different than the population norm.

2. Is your resting pressure in the normal range? How far is your systolic blood pressure from both borderline and isolated hypertension? How far is your diastolic blood pressure from mild, moderate, and severe hypertension? Describe two ways to decrease the risk of hypertension in your life.

3. What are your exercise blood pressure values? Are they within the normal range? What are your lab class exercise blood pressure values? Are they considered normal?

4. What aspect of blood pressure measurement do you think is most important to ensure accurate results? Why? Outline at least five additional variables that should be considered or controlled to ensure accurate blood pressure results.

Data Collection

Resting Blood Pressure

1. Each person in lab should practice measuring resting and exercise blood pressure.
2. Record the individual and class blood pressure results in Chart 4–4 and Chart 4–5, respectively. Compute the average blood pressures for the class.

Subjects should abide by the same preparatory guidelines that were outlined for HR measurement.

Resting Blood Pressure Measurement

1. Your partner should be seated with his or her *right arm* resting on the armrest of a chair or table. The upper arm should be at the approximate level of the heart.
2. To determine the appropriate cuff size, measure the circumference of your partner's upper arm. Based on this measurement select the proper cuff size as outlined in Table 4–2. *Note:* Avoid taking blood pressure readings over clothing. Sleeves should be rolled up. However, if the sleeve is rolled up and appears to fit tightly around the upper arm, remove the shirt or sweater, if possible.
3. Position the cuff so that the lower edge is approximately one inch (2.5 cm) above the antecubital space. The manometer should be clearly visible. If a mercury gauge is used, position it at eye level.

Table 4–2
Guidelines for Type of Blood Pressure Cuff

Upper Arm Circumference (at midpoint, cm)	Type of Cuff
Child	13 to 20 cm
Adult	17 to 26
Large Adult	32 to 42

Inflatable bladder width should be about 40% of the circumference of the arm; the length should be about 80% of the circumference of the arm.

Source: Pollock et al. (1990), and American Heart Association (1980).

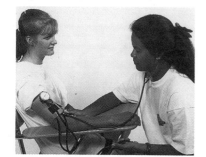

4. Insert the stethoscope ear tips directly down each ear canal. Gently tap the diaphragm to ensure suitable detection of sound.
5. Position the stethoscope diaphragm firmly over the brachial artery, in the antecubital space. If needed, palpate the brachial artery to find its location.
6. Tighten the air-release valve by turning it clockwise and quickly inflate the cuff to 150–160 mm Hg or to 20–30 mm Hg above the expected SBP. Inflating the cuff too much will cause unnecessary discomfort to your subject.
7. Turn the air-release valve counter-clockwise and release the cuff pressure at a *slow*, steady rate of about 2–5 mm Hg per second. *Note:* If you release it too fast you will be unable to distinguish the correct pressure at which the Korotkoff sounds appear or disappear. If you release it too slowly you may cause the subject excessive discomfort and apprehension.
8. Listen carefully and mentally note the pressure at which the Korotkoff sounds first appear (systolic blood pressure) and disappear (diastolic blood pressure).
9. Record your individual and class resting blood pressure values in Charts 4–4 and 4–5, respectively.
   Note: If a repeat blood pressure measurement is required for any reason, deflate the cuff completely. The pressure cuff must remain deflated for at least 10 seconds to allow the blood circulation to return to normal.

   The procedure for measuring blood pressure during both rest and exercise is essentially the same. It is rather easy to measure exercise blood pressure when your subject is riding a cycle ergometer. However, practice and experience is required to become skilled at blood pressure measurement during weight-bearing exercise such as treadmill jogging.

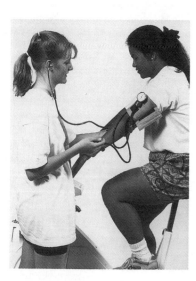

Exercise Blood Pressure Measurement

1. Have your partner exercise on a cycle ergometer (or other comparable alternative) at a moderate exercise intensity.
2. Measure exercise blood pressure during the final minute of a 3-minute bout of continuous exercise. If you choose to do weight-bearing exercise, measure blood pressure immediately post-exercise, after about 3 minutes of exercise.
3. Record the exercise blood pressure values in Charts 4–4 and 4–5, respectively.

HEART RATE AND BLOOD PRESSURE

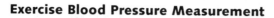

Name: _____   Date: _____

Measurement of Blood Pressure
Assignment

STATION 2

<table>
<tr><td colspan="3">Chart 4–4
Individual Blood Pressure Data Sheet</td></tr>
<tr><td></td><td>SBP
(mm Hg)</td><td>DBP
(mm Hg)</td></tr>
<tr><td>Resting</td><td></td><td></td></tr>
<tr><td>Exercise</td><td></td><td></td></tr>
</table>

	Chart 4–5 **Class Blood Pressure Data Sheet**			
	Resting		Exercise	
Subject	SPB (mm Hg)	DBP (mm Hg)	SBP (mm Hg)	DBP (mm Hg)
1				
2				
3				
4				
5				
6				
7				
8				
9				
10				
11				
12				
13				
14				
Class Total				
Class Average				

Research Conclusions

1. Is the average resting blood pressure in your laboratory class equal to the population average of 120/80 mm Hg? Describe at least two reasons why the lab average may be different than the population norm.

2. Is your resting pressure in the normal range? How far is your systolic blood pressure from both borderline and isolated hypertension? How far is your diastolic blood pressure from mild, moderate, and severe hypertension? Describe two ways to decrease the risk of hypertension in your life.

3. What are your exercise blood pressure values? Are they within the normal range? What are your lab class exercise blood pressure values? Are they considered normal?

4. What aspect of blood pressure measurement do you think is most important to ensure accurate results? Why? Outline at least five additional variables that should be considered or controlled to ensure accurate blood pressure results.

Name: _____ Date: _____

Lab 4 Summary

Describe several ways the information learned in this lab can be applied in your chosen field of interest and/or your personal life. Be specific and provide practical examples.

5

Cardiorespiratory Endurance
· ·
Pre-Laboratory Assignment

1. What is the predicted maximum oxygen consumption (expressed in $ml \cdot kg^{-1} \cdot min^{-1}$) of a 35-yr-old male who performs the step test? Assume he has a body weight of 180 lbs and a 15-second post-exercise pulse count of 32 beats. Record his age-adjusted VO_{2max} and fitness rating on the data sheet below.

2 a. What is the predicted maximum oxygen consumption (expressed in $L \cdot min^{-1}$) of a 23-yr-old female who performs the Astrand Cycle test? Assume the following data: body weight: 63 kg; ending heart rate: 144 bpm; ending work rate: 600 kgm/min.

VO_{2max} ($L \cdot min^{-1}$):_____(age corrected)

b. What is her age-corrected VO_{2max} expressed in $ml \cdot kg^{-1} \cdot min^{-1}$? Show work. Record her results on the data sheet below.

3. What is the predicted maximum oxygen consumption (expressed in $ml \cdot kg^{-1} \cdot min^{-1}$) of a 25-yr-old male who performs the George-Fisher jogging test? Assume he weighs 172 lbs, jogs the mile distance in 9:15 min:sec, and has an ending heart rate of 156 bpm. Show work and record results below.

Type of Test	VO_{2max} $(ml \cdot kg^{-1} \cdot min^{-1})$	Fitness Rating
Step test		
Astrand test		
George-Fisher jogging test		

4. ☐ Check the box if you have read each research question and are familiar with the data collection procedures regarding each research question.

5

Cardiorespiratory Endurance

PURPOSE

The purpose of this lab is to introduce you to several methods used to estimate cardiorespiratory endurance or maximal oxygen consumption (VO_{2max}).

STUDENT LEARNING OBJECTIVES

1. Be able to define cardiorespiratory endurance and explain how VO_{2max} is related to cardiorespiratory endurance and energy production.
2. Be able to describe how sub-maximal exercise tests estimate maximal cardiorespiratory endurance or aerobic capacity.
3. Learn how to effectively administer cardiorespiratory endurance prediction tests.

NECESSARY EQUIPMENT

Step benches
Cycle ergometers
Jogging or walking track
Metronome
Stop watches

PRE-LABORATORY PREPARATION

1. Wear comfortable exercise attire to class.
2. Avoid strenuous exercise at least 12 hours before testing.
3. Have no stimulants (tobacco, coffee, tea, colas, chocolate, etc.) nor depressants (alcohol, drugs, etc.) the day of the test.
4. Refrain from consuming a heavy meal within 3–4 hours before the laboratory class.

ASSESSMENT OF CARDIORESPIRATORY ENDURANCE

Cardiorespiratory endurance is the body's ability to sustain sub-maximal exercise for extended periods of time. Another common definition of cardiorespiratory endurance is the ability of the heart and vascular system to transport adequate amounts of oxygen to working muscles, allowing activities that involve large muscle masses, such as walking, running, or bicycling, to be performed over prolonged periods of time.

Cardiorespiratory endurance is a major component of physical fitness because it involves the pulmonary system for oxygen intake, cardiovascular system for oxygen and waste transport, and the muscular system for oxygen utilization. Consumption of oxygen is required for proper functioning of all the internal organs including the heart and brain.

Oxygen consumption has a positive linear relationship to energy production. As oxygen consumption increases, aerobic energy production increases to the point of maximal oxygen consumption (VO_{2max}) or maximal aerobic energy production.

Anaerobic energy, energy produced in the absence of oxygen, is quite limited and can be generated only for a few minutes during intense exercise. However, aerobic energy, energy produced in the presence of oxygen, can sustain exercise for several hours assuming sufficient amounts of foodstuffs are present in the cells.

Cardiorespiratory endurance is quantified in terms of maximal oxygen consumption (VO_{2max}) since the cardiovascular system is responsible for delivering oxygen to the active muscle. Cardiorespiratory endurance indirectly reflects a person's ability to perform aerobic activities and exercise. Can you describe the physiology of why individuals with heart disease have low levels of cardiorespiratory endurance? Conversely, can you see why marathon runners have high levels of cardiorespiratory endurance?

VO_{2max} is quantified in both absolute ($L \cdot min^{-1}$) and relative ($ml \cdot kg^{-1} \cdot min^{-1}$) terms. Both units can be used to indicate how hard the body is working during submaximal and/or maximal aerobic exertion. However, each unit value is used to express oxygen consumption and aerobic energy production for different reasons. The units *liters-per-minute* ($L \cdot min^{-1}$) represents the absolute or total amount of oxygen consumed in the body per minute. Absolute VO_{2max} is generally used to compute the total amount of aerobic energy or calories the body can generate.

Research has shown that approximately 5 kilocalories (kcal) of energy are produced for each liter of oxygen consumed (1 liter O_2 consumption = 5 kcals expended). For example:

$$\frac{4 \text{ liter } O_2}{min} \times \frac{5 \text{ kcal}}{1 \text{ liter } O_2} \approx \frac{20 \text{ kcal}}{min}$$

A kilocalorie (kcal) is defined as the amount of heat necessary to raise the temperature of 1 kg (1 liter) of water 1° C, from 14.5 to 15.5°C.

The units *milliliters of oxygen per kilogram per minute* ($ml \cdot kg^{-1} \cdot min^{-1}$), on the other hand, represent the rate of oxygen consumption required to move a kilogram of body weight per minute. VO_{2max} is most often expressed with relative units because a person's functional capacity is dependent on moving her own body weight.

In the human body, the total amount of oxygen consumed is important because it represents the total amount of energy available to do work. All else remaining equal, a person with a higher absolute VO_{2max} would be able to exercise at a higher intensity than a person with a lower VO_{2max}. However, because individuals have different body weights, expressing VO_{2max} in relative terms is more meaningful. For example, if two people have the same VO_{2max} of 4.5 $L \cdot min^{-1}$, but one person weighs 75 kg and the other 85 kg, then their relative VO_{2max} values will be 60 $ml \cdot kg^{-1} \cdot min^{-1}$ and 53 $ml \cdot kg^{-1} \cdot min^{-1}$, respectively. Even though both individuals have the same absolute capacity to consume and utilize oxygen, the 75 kg person has more oxygen available to move each unit of body weight than does the 85 kg person. Thus, the lighter person is able to

perform at a higher intensity or perform longer at a given intensity than his heavier counterpart, all else being equal. Can you see why obese individuals have low relative cardiorespiratory endurance levels? Can you see why athletes should lose excess body fat to maximize performance? Can you see the detrimental effects of a person gaining 25 pounds of fat weight? Normative data, based on relative VO_{2max} scores, is provided in Table 5–1.

Table 5–1
Cardiorespiratory Endurance Norm Chart
(VO$_{2max}$ values expressed in ml · kg^{-1} · min^{-1})

	Male				
Age	Poor	Fair	Average	Good	Excellent
<29	<25	25–33	34–42	43–52	>52
30–39	< 23	23–30	31–38	39–48	> 48
40–49	< 20	20–26	27–35	36–44	> 44
50–59	< 18	18–24	25–33	34–42	> 42
60–69	< 16	16–22	23–30	31–40	> 40
	Female				
<29	<24	24–30	31–37	38–48	>48
30–39	< 20	20–27	28–33	34–44	> 44
40–49	< 17	17–23	24–30	31–41	> 41
50–59	< 15	15–20	21–27	28–37	>37
60–69	<13	13–17	18–23	24–34	> 34

Source: American Heart Association (1972).

SELECTED REFERENCES

Adams, G. M. (1990). *Exercise Physiology Lab Manual.* Dubuque, Iowa: Wm. C. Brown Publishers, pp: 19–78.

American College of Sports Medicine (1991). *Guidelines of Exercise Testing and Prescription* (4th edition). Philadelphia: Lea & Febiger, pp: 39–43.

American Heart Association (1972). *Exercise Testing and Training of Apparently Healthy Individuals: A Handbook for Physicians.*, New York: p: 15.

Astrand, P.O., and I. Ryhming (1954). A nomogram for calculation of aerobic capacity (physical fitness) from pulse rate during submaximal work. *Journal of Applied Physiology* 7:218–221.

Cooper, K.H. (1968). A means of assessing maximal oxygen intake. *Journal of the American Medical Association* 203(3):135–138.

DeVries, H. A. (1986). *Physiology of Exercise: For Physical Education and Athletics* (4th edition). Dubuque, Iowa: Wm. C. Brown Publishers, pp: 210–218, 224–226, 266–278.

Fisher, A. G., and C. R. Jensen (1990). *Scientific Basis of Athletic Conditioning* (3rd edition). Philadelphia: Lea & Febiger, pp: 122–132, 251–254.

Fox, E. L., R. W. Bowers, and M. L. Foss (1988). *The Physiological Basis of Physical Education and Athletics* (4th edition). Philadelphia: Saunders College Publishing, pp: 61–67.

George, J. D., P. R. Vehrs, P. E. Allsen, G. W. Fellingham, and A. G. Fisher (1993). Development of a one-mile track jog for fit college aged individuals. *Medicine and Science in Sports and Exercise* 25(3):401–406.

Heyward, V. H., (1991). *Advanced Fitness Assessment and Exercise Prescription*. Champaign, Illinois: Human Kinetic Books, pp: 17–69.

Hoeger, W. W. K. (1989). *Lifetime Physical Fitness and Wellness: A Personalized Program*. Englewood, Colorado: Morton Publishing Company, pp:15–41.

Howley, E. T., and D. B. Frank (1992). *Health Fitness Instructor's Handbook* (2nd edition). Champaign, Illinois: Human Kinetics, pp: 35–45, 153–177.

Kline, G. M., J. P. Porcari, R. Hintermeister, et al. (1987). Estimation of VO_{2max} from a one-mile track walk, gender, age, and body weight. *Medicine and Science in Sports and Exercise* 19(3):253–259.

Lamb, D. R. (1984). *Physiology of Exercise: Responses and Adaptations* (2nd edition). New York: Macmillan Publishing Company, pp: 99–103, 173–190.

McArdle, W. D., F. I. Katch, and V. L. Katch (1991). *Exercise Physiology: Energy, Nutrition, and Human Performance* (3rd edition). Philadelphia: Lea & Febiger, pp: 211–232.

Noble, B. J. (1986). *Physiology of Exercise and Sport*. St. Louis, Missouri: Times Mirror/Mosby College Publishing, pp: 96–111, 122–123, 229–256.

Powers, S. K., and E. T. Howley (1990). *Exercise Physiology: Theory and Application to Fitness and Performance*. Dubuque, Iowa: Wm. C. Brown Publishers, pp: 117–130, 303–328, 428–430.

Siconolfi, S. F., E. M. Cullinane, R. A. Carleton, and R. D. Thompson (1982). Assessing VO_{2max} in epidemiologic studies: modification of the Astrand-Ryhming test. *Medicine and Science in Sport and Exercise* 14(5):335–338.

Sharkey, B. J. (1977). *Fitness and Work Capacity* (Report FS-315). Washington, DC: U.S. Department of Agriculture, Department of Forest Service.

Sharkey, B. J. (1991). *Physiology of Fitness*. , Champaign, Illinois: Human Kinetics.

Washburn, R. A., and M. J. Safrit (1982). Physical performance tests in job selection—a model for empirical validation. *Research Quarterly for Exercise and Sport* 53(3):267–270.

Wilmore, J. H., and D. L. Costill (1988). *Training for Sport and Activity: The Physiological Basis of the Conditioning Process* (3rd edition). Dubuque, Iowa: Wm. C. Brown Publishers, pp: 367–369.

STATION 1

. . . .

Forest Service Step Test

Research Questions

1. Do you meet the minimal cardiorespiratory endurance requirements to work for the U.S. Forest Service? Past experience has shown that employees require a minimum VO_{2max} of 45 ml·kg^{-1}·min^{-1}. Are you within 10% of this criterion minimum? Show your work.

2. Does this appear to be an acceptable test for the Forest Service to use for screening fire-fighting job applicants? Defend your answer.

3. What other parameter(s) of physical fitness may be important for fighting fires? Explain. Should these parameters be included when screening job applicants? Why?

4. Describe at least two advantages and disadvantages to the step test.

Data Collection

The *Forest Service Step Test* requires one to perform repetitive bench stepping for a period of 5 minutes. Cardiorespiratory endurance is predicted based on gender, work rate, heart rate, body weight, and age. (An alternative step test can be substituted for the *Forest Service Step Test* if your lab has another preference.)

1. Set the metronome to a cadence of 90 beats per minute (22.5 step cycles per minute).
2. Men: Use a bench that is 15 inches tall.
   Women: Use a bench that is 13 inches tall.
3. Begin the step test by stepping onto and down from the bench in cadence with the metronome. Every four beats of the metronome represents one complete stepping cycle. Each beat of the metronome represents a single step as follows:
   a. Step up onto the bench with your right foot.
   b. Step up onto the bench with your left foot.
   c. Step down from the bench with your right foot.
   d. Step down from the bench with your left foot.
      Your leading foot may be changed a few times during the test. Be sure to straighten your legs at the top of each step.
4. Perform the step test for 5 minutes.
5. At the end of 5 minutes, immediately sit down and have your partner palpate your pulse.
6. Sit quietly for 15 seconds.
7. Measure a 15-second pulse count between the 15th and 30th second

following the 5-minute test. Be sure to turn off the metronome so it does not interfere with the counting of your pulse. Record the number of heart beats in Chart 5–1.

8. After the pulse count measurement, a cool-down period of slow walking or static stretching is advised.

9. Use your body weight and 15-second post-exercise pulse count to determine your fitness score in $ml \cdot kg^{-1} \cdot min^{-1}$ from Table 5–2 if you are male, or Table 5–3 if you are female. Find your pulse count in the far left column of the table. Note that body weight values are positioned along the bottom of the tables. Read horizontally from your pulse count value until you reach the column that contains your body weight. The value that is at the intersection of the pulse count row and the body weight column is your non-adjusted VO_{2max} in $ml \cdot kg^{-1} \cdot min^{-1}$.

10. Obtain your age correction factor from Table 5–4. Multiply your non-adjusted VO_{2max} from Table 5–2 or 5–3 times your age correction factor. The result equals your age-adjusted fitness score, or your estimated VO_{2max}.

11. Record your age-adjusted VO_{2max} in Chart 5–1.

12. Compute your absolute aerobic capacity in $L \cdot min^{-1}$ and record it in Chart 5–1.

13. Determine your fitness rating from the cardiorespiratory norm chart (Table 5-1) and record it in Chart 5–1.

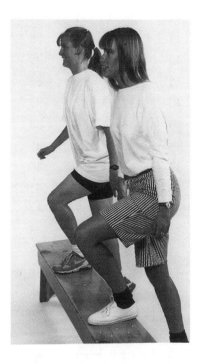

Computation Example: A 46-year-old female subject has a body weight of 130 pounds (58.9 kg) and a 15-second post-exercise pulse count of 26 beats. What is her cardiorespiratory endurance in both $ml \cdot kg^{-1} \cdot min^{-1}$ and $L \cdot min^{-1}$?

1. Her non-adjusted fitness score from Table 5–3 is 51 $ml \cdot kg^{-1} \cdot min^{-1}$.

2. The age correction factor from Table 5–4 is 0.91. Thus her age-adjusted score is:

$$51 \ ml \cdot kg^{-1} min^{-1} \times 0.91 = 46.4 \ ml \cdot kg^{-1} \cdot min^{-1}$$

3. The cardiorespiratory endurance in $L \cdot min^{-1}$ is computed as follows:

$$46.4 \ \frac{ml/min}{kg} \times 58.9 \ kg = 2733.5 \ ml/min$$

$$2733.5 \ \frac{ml}{min} \times \frac{1 \ liter}{1000 \ m} = 2.73 \ \frac{liters}{min}$$

4. A cardiorespiratory endurance score of 46.4 $ml \cdot kg^{-1} \cdot min^{-1}$ for a 46-year-old female is in the Excellent category based on the norms in Table 5–1.

Table 5–2
Forestry Step Test for Men

(Non-adjusted VO$_{2max}$ estimations (ml·kg^{-1}·min^{-1})

15 Second
Pulse Count

	120	130	140	150	160	170	180	190	200	210	220	230	240
44	34	34	34	34	33	33	33	33	33	33	33	33	33
43	35	35	35	34	34	34	34	34	34	34	34	34	34
42	36	35	35	35	35	35	35	35	35	35	35	35	35
41	36	36	36	36	36	36	36	36	36	36	36	36	36
40	37	37	37	37	37	37	37	37	37	37	37	37	37
39	38	38	38	38	38	38	38	38	38	38	38	37	37
38	39	39	39	39	39	39	39	39	39	39	39	38	38
37	41	40	40	40	40	40	40	40	40	40	40	39	39
36	42	42	41	41	41	41	41	41	41	41	41	40	40
35	43	43	42	42	42	42	42	42	42	42	42	42	41
34	44	44	43	43	43	43	43	43	43	43	43	43	43
33	46	45	45	45	45	45	44	44	44	44	44	44	44
32	47	47	46	46	46	46	46	46	46	46	46	46	46
31	48	48	48	47	47	47	47	47	47	47	47	47	47
30	50	49	49	49	49	48	48	48	48	48	48	48	48
29	52	51	51	51	50	50	50	50	50	50	50	50	50
28	53	53	53	53	52	52	52	52	52	51	51	51	51
27	55	55	55	54	54	54	54	54	54	53	53	53	52
26	57	57	56	56	56	56	56	56	56	55	55	54	54
25	59	59	58	58	58	58	58	58	58	56	56	55	55
24	60	60	60	60	60	60	60	59	59	58	58	57	
23	62	62	61	61	61	61	61	60	60	60	59		
22	64	64	63	63	63	63	62	62	61	61			
21	66	66	65	65	65	64	64	64	62				
20	68	68	67	67	67	67	66	66	65				

Body Weight (lbs)

Source: Sharkey (1991).

Table 5–3
Forestry Step Test for Women

(Non-adjusted VO$_{2max}$ estimations (ml·kg^{-1}·min^{-1})

15 Second
Pulse Count

	80	90	100	110	120	130	140	150	160	170	180	190
44								30	30	30	30	30
43							31	31	31	31	31	31
42			32	32	32	32	32	32	32	32	32	32
41			33	33	33	33	33	33	33	33	33	33
40			34	34	34	34	34	34	34	34	34	34
39			35	35	35	35	35	35	35	35	35	35
38			36	36	36	36	36	36	36	36	36	36
37			37	37	37	37	37	37	37	37	37	37
36		37	38	38	38	38	38	38	38	38	38	38
35	38	38	39	39	39	39	39	39	39	39	39	39
34	39	39	40	40	40	40	40	40	40	40	40	40
33	40	40	41	41	41	41	41	41	41	41	41	41
32	41	41	42	42	42	42	42	42	42	42	42	42
31	42	42	43	43	43	43	43	43	43	43	43	43
30	43	43	44	44	44	44	44	44	44	44	44	44
29	44	44	45	45	45	45	45	45	45	45	45	45
28	45	45	46	46	46	47	47	47	47	47	47	47
27	46	46	47	48	48	49	49	49	49	49		
26	47	48	49	50	50	51	51	51	51			
25	49	50	51	52	52	53	53					
24	51	52	53	54	54	55						
23	53	54	55	56	56	57						

Body Weight (lbs)

Source: Sharkey (1991).

Table 5–4
Age-Correction Factors

Age	c.f.
15	1.04
20	1.02
25	1.00
30	0.97
35	0.95
40	0.93
45	0.91
50	0.88
55	0.86
60	0.82
65	0.80

Modified from Sharkey (1991).

Name: _____   Date: _____

Cardiorespiratory Endurance
Assignment

Age: _____   Gender: M   F

Body Weight: _____ lbs   _____ kg

STATION 1

Chart 5–1
Forest Service Step Test **Data Sheet**
Heart Rate Data: Palpate your pulse from the 15th to the 30th second following the 5-minute step test. Post-Exercise Pulse Count: _____ beats per 15 seconds
Predicted Cardiovascular Endurance (VO_{2max}): Age correction factor: _____ Non-adjusted predicted VO_{2max}: _____ $ml \cdot kg^{-1} \cdot min^{-1}$ Age-adjusted predicted VO_{2max}: _____ $ml \cdot kg^{-1} \cdot min^{-1}$ Age-adjusted predicted VO_{2max}: _____ $L \cdot min^{-1}$ Cardiorespiratory endurance fitness rating: _____

For age correction factor, see Table 5–4.

For non-adjusted predicted VO_{2max}, see Table 5–2 or 5–3.

Age-adjusted predicted VO_{2max} = Non-adjusted score × correction factor

Research Conclusions

1. Do you meet the minimal cardiorespiratory endurance requirements to work for the U.S. Forest Service? Past experience has shown that employees require a minimum VO_{2max} of 45 ml·kg^{-1}·min^{-1}. Are you within 10% of this criterion measure? Show your work.

2. Does this appear to be an acceptable test for the Forest Service to use for screening fire-fighting job applicants? Defend your answer.

3. What other parameter(s) of physical fitness may be important for fighting fires? Explain. Should these parameters be included when screening job applicants? Why?

4. Describe at least two advantages and disadvantages to the step test.

STATION 2
. . . .
Astrand Cycle Test

Research Questions

1. What is your estimated VO_{2max} for the Astrand Cycle Test? What is your fitness category based on the results of this test?

2. What is your estimated maximum caloric expenditure (kcal/min) based on the results of this test? Assume 1 liter O_2 consumed = 5 kcal expended.

3. If you could ride a cycle ergometer at 70% of your VO_{2max}, how many minutes would it take to expend 300 kcals?

4. If you could ride at 85% of your VO_{2max} instead of 70%, how many fewer minutes would it take to expend 300 kcals? Discuss the implications of your findings.

Data Collection

The *Astrand Cycle Test* involves riding a stationary bicycle for approximately six minutes. The exercise intensity is sub-maximal and relatively easy for most people to perform. The prediction of cardiorespiratory endurance (VO_{2max}) is based on a person's gender, age, exercise heart rate, and ergometer work rate. As the work rate increases during the test, oxygen consumption and energy production increases. In order to transport essential oxygen to the working tissues, the heart is stimulated to beat at a higher rate. Research has demonstrated that work rate, oxygen consumption, and heart rate have a direct, positive relationship to cardiorespiratory endurance (VO_{2max}). In fact, the relationship is most linear between 50 and 85% maximal heart rate (HR_{max}).

To quantify cardiorespiratory endurance based on a given exercise heart rate response, it is also necessary to know the exercise work rate. Work rate is calculated using the following formula:

$$\text{Work rate (power)} = \frac{\text{force} \times \text{distance}}{\text{time}} \text{ or force} \times \frac{\text{revolution}}{\text{min}} \times \frac{\text{meter}}{\text{revolution}}$$

For the cycle ergometer, force is modified by adjusting the tension of the belt around the flywheel. Distance on the Monarch ergometer is 6 meters per revolution since each time a given pedal makes one complete revolution the flywheel travels (rotates) 6 meters. The *time* component is used to determine the rate and depends on how many revolutions are completed per unit time. A metronome or rpm gauge is typically used to quantify the pedal rate.

To illustrate, at the end of the Astrand Cycle Test a subject was exercising at the following work rates:

$$\text{Force} = 3.5 \text{ kg}$$
$$\text{Distance} = 6 \text{ meters/revolution of the bicycle flywheel}$$
$$\text{Time} = 50 \text{ revolutions/minute}$$
$$\text{Work rate} = 3.5 \text{ kg} \times 6 \text{ m/rev} \times 50 \text{ rev/min}$$
$$\text{Work rate} = 1050 \text{ kgm} \cdot \text{min}^{-1}$$

The computed work rate is then used to predict VO_{2max}. Follow the procedures below for the Astrand Cycle Test. Record your data in Chart 5–2.

1. Pair up in groups of two. Calculate your predicted HR_{max} based on the simple regression equation: 220 minus age. Record your results in Chart 5–2.

2. Calculate 60% and 70% of your age-predicted HR_{max} and corresponding 15-second pulse counts. For example:

   Predicted $HR_{max} \times 0.60 = 60\% \ HR_{max}$
   Predicted $HR_{max} \times 0.70 = 70\% \ HR_{max}$
   $60\% \ HR_{max} \div 4 = $ 15-second pulse count for $60\% \ HR_{max}$
   $70\% \ HR_{max} \div 4 = $ 15-second pulse count for $70\% \ HR_{max}$

3. Adjust the cycle ergometer seat height so that your knees are almost fully extended when the pedals are at their lowest point. Be sure to cycle with your toes on the pedals. The seat is generally at the correct height if the leg is straight when the heel of the foot is positioned on the pedal at its lowest point. Record the seat height in Chart 5–2.

4. If using a metronome, set the cadence at 100 bpm. A 100 bpm setting is equivalent to a pedal rate of 50 revolutions per minute, if on each beat of the metronome, one pedal is at the bottom of a given down stroke.

5. Once you have achieved the proper cadence, have your partner set the resistance to the prescribed workload from the protocol as outlined in Table 5–5. Your partner is to measure your exercise heart rate at each workload and record this information on your data sheet.

6. Begin timing each stage after the work rate is properly set.

7. Cycle at each work rate for 2 minutes. Have your partner measure your 15-second pulse within the last 30 seconds of each 2-minute stage and record your work rate and 15-second heart rate on Chart 5–2. Increase the workload after each stage as indicated in Table 5–6 or 5–7. Continue the test until you reach a workload that elicits a pulse count ≥ 70% of age-predicted HR_{max}.

8. At the completion of the test, record your ending work rate and final 15-second heart rate in Chart 5–2.

9. Decrease the workload of the ergometer to a comfortable level and cool down for 2–3 minutes.

10. Convert each 15-second heart rate to beats per minute (bpm).

Table 5–5
Common Work Rates for Astrand Test

Force (kg)	Speed* (m·min⁻¹)	Work Rate† (kgm·min⁻¹)
0.5	300	150
1.0	300	300
1.5	300	450
2.0	300	600
2.5	300	750
3.0	300	900
3.5	300	1050
4.0	300	1200

*Speed: 50 rpm × 6 meters/rev = 300 meters/min
†Work Rate: Force × Speed

11. Using the Astrand nomogram (Figure 5–1), determine your non-adjusted aerobic capacity (L·min⁻¹) from your ending work rate and heart rate (bpm). (See the example below.) Record your results in Chart 5–2.

Table 5–6

Astrand Protocol for Women and Men Over Age 35

Beginning workload: 0.5 kg (150 kgm·min⁻¹)

Pedal speed: 50 rpm

Time of each stage: 2 minutes

During the last 30 seconds of each stage, measure a 15-second pulse.

If HR is < 70% HR_{max}, increase the workload by 0.5 kg and continue pedaling for another 2 minutes. Repeat step one.

If HR is ≥ 70% HR_{max}, do *not* increase the work load and continue pedaling until steady-state heart rate is reached.

Source: Siconolfi (1982).

Table 5–7

Astrand Protocol for Men Under Age 35

Beginning workload: 1 kg (300 kgm·min⁻¹)

Pedal speed: 50 rpm

Time of each stage: 2 minutes

During the last 30 seconds of each stage, measure a 15-second pulse.

If HR is < 70% HR_{max}, increase the workload by 1.0 kg and continue pedaling for another 2 minutes. Repeat step one.

If HR is ≥ 70% HR_{max}, do *not* increase the work load and continue pedaling until steady-state heart rate is reached.

Source: Siconolfi (1982).

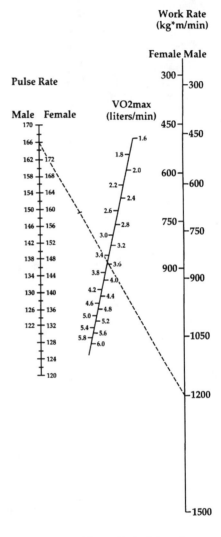

Figure 5–1. Astrand nomogram.

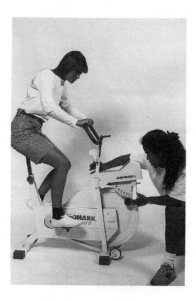

12. Multiply your non-adjusted VO_{2max} value by the proper age-correction factor from Table 5–4 to correct your VO_{2max} value for age. Record your age-adjusted VO_{2max} value on Chart 5–2.

13. Convert your age-adjusted VO_2max value from $L \cdot min^{-1}$ to $ml \cdot kg^{-1}min^{-1}$. (See the example below.)

14. Determine your fitness rating from the norm chart (Table 5–1) and record it on Chart 5–2.

Computation Example: A 21-year-old male has an ending workload of 1200 $kgm \cdot min^{-1}$ and an ending heart rate of 166 $beats \cdot min^{-1}$. What is his predicted VO_{2max} in $ml \cdot kg^{-1} \cdot min^{-1}$? Assume he has a body weight of 80 kg.

1. In the Astrand nomogram (Figure 5–1), notice the dashed line example. This line was drawn with a straight edge from the male heart rate mark of 166 bpm over to the male work rate mark of 1200 $kgm \cdot min^{-1}$. Notice the dashed line intersects the VO_{2max} line at the 3.6 $L \cdot min^{-1}$. mark. This value of 3.6 $L \cdot min^{-1}$ is the subject's non-adjusted VO_{2max}.

2. Multiply the non-adjusted VO_{2max} times the age correction factor in (Table 5–4) to determine the age-adjusted VO_{2max} score.

$$3.6 \ L \cdot min^{-1} \times 1.02 = 3.67$$

3. Convert the adjusted value ($l \cdot min^{-1}$) to $ml \cdot kg^{-1} \cdot min^{-1}$.

$$\frac{3.67 \ L/min \ \times 1000 \ ml/L}{80 \ kg} = 45.8 \ ml \cdot kg^{-1} \cdot min^{-1}$$

4. Determine his fitness rating on the norm chart (Table 5–1). His cardiovascular endurance rating is good.

Notes:

1. During the final workload, steady-state heart rate is realized when two sequential 15-second pulse counts are within 1 beat of one another.

2. Continue pedaling (at 50 rpm) when pulse counts are palpated and\or between stages until the final workload is attained.

3. The test is terminated at a workload that elicits a steady state heart rate $\geq$ 70% age predicted HR_{max}.

4. Palpate your partner's pulse at the radial artery or carotid artery. Press gently to prevent occlusion of blood flow.

Name: _____ Date: _____

Astrand Cycle Test
Assignment

STATION 2

Chart 5–2
Astrand Cycle Test Data Sheet

Pre-Test Heart Rate Data

Seat Height: _____9_____

Age-predicted maximum HR (220–age): ___20/___ bpm

Age correction factor: _____

60% of HR_{max}: ___120.6___ bpm   15-second pulse: ___30,15___

70% of HR_{max}: ___140,7___ bpm   15-second pulse: ___35,175___

Work Rate and Heart Rate Data			
Time (min)	Work Rate (kgm · min^{-1})	Heart Rate (15-second)	Heart Rate (beats · min^{-1})
0–2			
2–4			
4–6			
6–8			
8–10			

Predicted Cardiorespiratory Endurance:

VO_{2max}: _____ L·min^{-1} (See Figure 5–1)

VO_{2max}: _____ L·min^{-1} (Age-adjusted)

VO_{2max}: _____ ml·kg^{-1}·min^{-1}

Cardiorespiratory Endurance Rating: _____

Research Conclusions

1. What is your estimated VO$_{2max}$ for the Astrand Cycle Test? What is your fitness category based on the results of this test?

2. What is your estimated maximum caloric expenditure (kcal/min) based on the results of this test? Assume 1 liter O$_2$ consumed = 5 kcal expended.

3. If you could ride a bicycle at 70% of your VO$_{2max}$, how many minutes would you need to exercise in order to expend 300 kcals?

4. If you could ride at 85% of your VO$_{2max}$ instead of 70%, how many fewer minutes would it take to expend 300 kcals? Discuss the implications of your findings

STATION 3
Rockport Walking Test and George-Fisher Jogging Test

Research Questions

1. Do walking and jogging tests predict cardiorespiratory endurance to within ± 5 ml·kg^{-1}·min^{-1} of one another? Explain why the two tests should generate similar results and why they might generate different results.

2. Describe at least two reasons why it might be of value to have access to both a walking and jogging test to evaluate cardiorespiratory endurance?

3. Do you think college fitness courses should use submaximal exercise tests (i.e., walking and/or jogging protocols) instead of the maximal performance tests such as the 1.5 mile run? Justify your answer.

Data Collection

Station 3 can be used as a take-home assignment when there is insufficient time to complete these tests during class time.

Rockport Walking Test

The Rockport Walking Test is a simple, self-paced test that almost anyone who can walk is capable of performing. The test protocol requires a person walk a mile as quickly as possible and then measure his heart rate and walking time. A regression equation has been developed that allows estimation of cardiorespiratory endurance based on the 1-mile walk test results.

Instructions (Kline et al., 1987):

1. On a measured track, walk one mile as fast as possible. Walk on the inside lane when using a standard multi-lane track. When finished, record the time of the walk to the nearest minute and hundredth minute. Record this information in Chart 5–3.
2. Measure your 10-second immediate post-exercise pulse following the mile walk. Record the information in Chart 5–3.
3. Using the regression equation outlined below, compute your relative fitness level.
4. Determine your cardiorespiratory fitness classification using the norm chart (Table 5-1). Record your results in Chart 5–3.

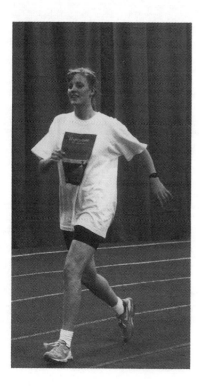

$$VO_{2max} = 132.6 - (0.17 \times Wt) - (0.39 \times Age) + (6.31 \times G) - (3.27 \times T)$$
$$-(0.156 \times HR)$$

Where: $VO_{2max} = ml \cdot kg^{-1} \cdot min^{-1}$.

        Wt $=$ Body weight (kg)

        Age $=$ Age in years

    Gender(G) $=$ 0 for female and 1 for male

    Time (T) $=$ Time to walk 1 mile (00:00)

        HR $=$ Palpated post-exercise heart rate (bpm)

Computation Example: A 30-year-old male weighing 68.2 kg performs the 1-mile walk in 12:35 min:sec. What is his cardiorespiratory endurance in $ml \cdot kg^{-1} \cdot min^{-1}$? Assume that he measures a 10-second post-exercise heart rate of 20 beats immediately following the exercise.

1. Convert his walk time from a 00:00 value to a 00.00 value. This must be done to allow for a numerical computation within the regression equation below.

   The walk time of 12:35 is converted to a 00.00 value by changing the 35-second figure to a decimal. This is done by dividing 35 by 60.

   $$35 \sec onds \times \frac{1\, minute}{60\, seconds} = 0.58\, minutes$$

   Thus the 12:35 test time is 12.58 minutes.

2. Convert the heart rate data to a minute rate. For example:

   $$\frac{20\, beats}{10\, seconds} \times \frac{60\, seconds}{1\, minute} = 120\, bpm$$

3. Compute the person's predicted VO_{2max} (aerobic capacity) using the following regression equation:

   $$VO_{2max} = 132.6 - (0.17 \times Wt) - (0.39 \times Age) + (6.31 \times G)$$
   $$- (3.27 \times T) - (0.156 \times HR)$$

   $$VO_{2max} = 132.6 - (0.17 \times 68.2) - (0.39 \times 30) + (6.31 \times 1)$$
   $$- (3.27 \times 12.58) - (0.156 \times 120)$$

   $$VO_{2max} = 55.77 \; ml \cdot kg^{-1} \cdot min^{-1}$$

4. Fitness Level: Excellent (See Table 5–1).

George-Fisher Jogging Test

The George-Fisher Jogging Test is a cardiorespiratory fitness test designed to serve as a submaximal alternative for the 1.5-mile run, an all-out distance run. The equipment and data collection needs for the jogging test are similar to that of the walking test. A regression equation has been developed that estimates a person's cardiorespiratory endurance based on exercise heart rate, jog time, gender, and body weight. Research has recently demonstrated that a 1-mile track jog can estimate cardiorespiratory endurance (VO_{2max}) as well as the 1.5-mile run.

Instructions:

1. Jog one mile at a steady, moderate pace. Because this test requires jogging at a relatively slow speed, the following criteria must be met to maintain the accuracy of the test.

   Pre-test tip: Prior to the test, jog a single lap around the track at a comfortable pace. Record your time. If it is above the lowest allowable time listed above, that pace is suitable for the test. If your warm-up jogging speed and heart rate are appropriate, proceed with the 1-mile jogging test. Be sure to maintain the same jogging speed during the entire mile distance; never speed up or slow down at any time.

   Speed criteria: Males must jog the mile distance in an elapsed time of at least 8:00 minutes or more. Females must jog the mile in at least 9:00 minutes or more. If you jog the mile in less than the allotted time, rest and then perform the test again at a slower speed. On a 440-yard track the lowest acceptable time would be 2 minutes per lap for males and 2:15 minutes for females.

   Heart rate criteria: 180 bpm is the upper limit. At the end of the mile if your heart rate is elevated above 180 bpm, rest and then perform the test again at a slower speed.

2. Immediately after the jog, measure a 10-second post-exercise pulse.
3. Record the elapsed jog time in minutes:seconds.
4. Record your pulse count and the elapsed time in Chart 5–3.
5. Using the following regression equation, compute your relative fitness level (George et al. 1993). Show your work.

$$VO_{2max} = 100.5 + (8.344 \times G) - (0.1636 \times Wt) - (1.438 \times T) - (0.1928 \times HR)$$

Where: $VO_{2max} = ml \cdot kg^{-1} \cdot min^{-1}$

   Wt = Body weight (kg)

   Gender(G) = 0 for female; 1 for male

   Time (T) = Time to jog 1 mile (00:00)

   HR = Palpated post-exercise heart rate (bpm)

6. Determine your cardiorespiratory fitness classification from Table 5–1.

   Note that the 1-mile jog test was developed for individuals aged 18–29 years old. If you are ≥ 30 years old, age-adjust your estimated VO_{2max} score with a factor found in Table 5–4.

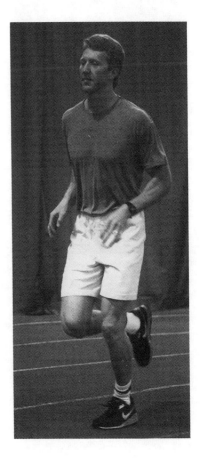

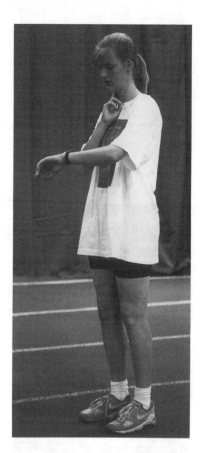

Computation Example: Suppose a college female weighing 65.4 kg performs the 1-mile jogging test in 9:47 min:sec. What is her cardiorespiratory endurance (VO_{2max}) in ml·kg^{-1}·min^{-1}? Assume that she measures a post-exercise heart rate of 27 beats within 10 seconds immediately following the exercise.

1. Convert her jog time from a 00:00 value to a 00.00 value. This must be done to allow for a numerical computation within the regression equation below. The jog time of 9:47 is converted to a 00.00 value by changing the 47 second figure to a decimal. This is done by dividing 47 by 60.

$$47 \text{ seconds} \times \frac{1 \text{ minute}}{60 \text{ seconds}} = 0.78 \text{ minutes}$$

Thus the 9:47 test time is 9.78 minutes.

2. Convert the heart rate data to a bpm rate. For example:

$$\frac{27 \text{ beats}}{10 \text{ seconds}} \times \frac{60 \text{ seconds}}{1 \text{ minute}} = 162 \text{ bpm}$$

3. Compute this person's predicted VO_{2max} (aerobic capacity) using the following regression equation:

$$VO_{2max} = 100.5 + (8.344 \times G) - (0.1636 \times Wt) - (1.438 \times T) - (0.1928 \times HR)$$

$$VO_{2max} \text{ (ml·kg}^{-1}\text{·min}^{-1}) = 100.5 + (8.344 \times 0) - (0.1636 \times 65.4) - (1.438 \times 9.78) - (0.1928 \times 162)$$

$$VO_{2max} = 44.5 \text{ ml·kg}^{-1}\text{·min}^{-1}$$

Fitness Level: Good (See Table 5–1).

Astrand Cycle Test
Assignment

STATION 3

Chart 5–3
Walking & Jogging Test Protocols
Data Sheet

Rockport Walking Test Results:

1-mile jog time: _____ min:sec (00.00)

1-mile walk time: _____ minutes (00.00)

10-sec post-exercise pulse count: _____ beats

Post-exercise pulse rate: _____ beats/minute

Cardiovascular Endurance Results:

$VO_2max = 132.6 - (0.17 \times Wt) - (0.39 \times Age) + (6.31 \times G) - (3.27 \times T) - (0.156 \times HR)$

VO_{2max}: _____ $ml \cdot kg^{-1} \cdot min^{-1}$

Cardiorespiratory Endurance Rating: _____

George-Fisher Jogging Test Results:

1-mile jog time: _____ min: sec (00:00)

1-mile jog time: _____ minutes (00:00)

10-sec post-exercise pulse count: _____ beats

Post-exercise pulse rate: _____ beats/minute

Cardiovascular Endurance Results:

$VO_{2max} = 100.5 + (8.344 \times G) - (0.1636 \times Wt) - (1.438 \times T) - (0.1928 \times HR)$

VO_{2max}: _____ $ml \cdot kg^{-1} \cdot min^{-1}$

Cardiorespiratory Endurance Rating: _____

Research Conclusions

1. Do walking and jogging tests predict cardiorespiratory endurance to within ± 5 ml·kg⁻¹·min⁻¹ of one another? Explain why the two tests should generate similar results and why they might generate different results.

2. Describe at least two reasons why it might be of value to have access to both a walking and jogging test to evaluate cardiovascular endurance?

3. Do you think college fitness courses should use submaximal exercise tests (i.e., walking and/or jogging protocols) instead of the maximal performance tests such as the 1.5-mile run? Justify your answer.

Name: _____ Date: _____

Lab 5 Summary

Describe several ways the information learned in this lab can be applied in your chosen field of interest and/or your personal life. Be specific and provide practical examples.

6

Body Composition
. . . .
Pre-Laboratory Assignment

1. What is the height-squared index of a six-foot female? What is her predicted percent fat assuming she weighs 100 kg? Show your work.

2. A 5'10", 25-year-old, 93 kg male has a waist measurement of 42 inches and a hip measurement of 36 inches. What is his body mass index and waist-to-hip ratio?

3. A 69-inch female has a waist and hip circumference measurement of 89 cm and 114.3 cm, respectively. What is her predicted percent body fat? Show your work.

4. A 45-year-old male subject is measured to have a three-skinfolds sum of 45 mm. What is his predicted body density and estimated percent fat? Show your work.

5. ☐ Check the box if you have read each research question and are familiar with the data collection procedures regarding each research question.

6

Body Composition

Body composition refers to the composition of the various components of the human body. In exercise science there are two major components of the body that are of interest: fat-free mass (lean body mass: muscle, bone, organs, water, etc.) and fat mass. A person with a high amount of lean body mass compared to fat mass is considered lean. Conversely, a person who carries excess body fat compared to fat-free mass is considered obese. A body composition evaluation can provide valuable information about both of these two important components of the human body.

The body composition of an individual directly affects the ability to move. For instance, while very important to the human organism, fat weight is non-contractile tissue and therefore detrimental to body movement in many aspects of life such as daily activity, recreational games, and athletic competition. Skeletal muscle, on the other hand, is beneficial since it is contractile tissue that serves to move the body. In terms of weight-bearing exercise, a person can maximize performance if a proper balance between lean and fat weight can be realized. For example, a male who weighs 200 pounds and has 15 percent body fat (%BF) would be able to function better than a 200-pound male with 30% BF. The leaner male would have relatively more muscle mass to move his body as compared to the fatter male.

It is misleading to think that a body free of fat is ideal, even for the athlete. The human body requires some fat to function properly and essential fat typically represents about 3–5% of body weight for males and 10–14% for females.

There are several practical reasons for measuring body composition.

1. Some individuals think they are obese when they really are not; conversely, some think they are lean when in actuality the reverse is true. A body composition test, if accurate, can tell a person whether or not a composition problem exists that needs to be addressed.

2. Based on the results of a body composition test, a prudent plan for improvement or maintenance can be outlined. Accordingly, goals can be set that are realistic and achievable.

3. Improvements and/or regressions in a person's body composition status can be monitored over time to track progress. Such knowledge can provide the impetus for continued participation in exercise programs.

For many individuals, the relationship between body weight and body fat is positive, i.e., as body weight increases, body fat increases. However there are exceptions to this general relationship. For instance, certain individuals who increase their lean tissue (muscle or bone) through regular, strenuous exercise often display an inverse relationship between body weight and body fat. In addition, thin, sedentary individuals who have a low body weight, yet relatively high amounts of fat also confound the body weight to body fat relationship. Such individuals may appear lean and in shape but have atrophied muscle and excessive fat due to lack of exercise and/or poor dietary habits.

Because body weight measures can be very misleading, body composition tests are recommended when monitoring the effects of physical training or nutrition modification. Body weight measures by themselves are ineffective when monitoring changes in body composition since decreases in weight are not always indicative of decreases in body fat, and an increase in weight may be the result of an increase in muscle mass. Is it clear why weight scales are an invalid measure of body fat and ineffective when monitoring changes in body composition?

There are many different types of tests that predict or estimate percent body fat. Prediction tests are generally quick and relatively easy to perform, inexpensive, and used for the mass testing of large groups of people. Such advantages are very appealing in many health and fitness settings. However, prediction tests are inherently less accurate than hydrostatic weighing, assuming both tests are properly administered.

HYDROSTATIC WEIGHING

Hydrostatic weighing is based on principles of densitometry, the measurement of body density. The underlying basis for this method is that body density is

Table 6–1
Body Composition Classification According to Percent Body Fat

Age	Ideal	Good	Moderate	Fat	Obese
Men					
<19	12	12.5–17.0	17.5–22.0	22.5–27.0	27.5+
20–29	13	13.5–18.0	18.5–23.0	23.5-28.0	28.5+
30–39	14	14.5–19.0	19.5–24.0	24.5–29.0	29.5+
40–49	15	15.5–20.0	20.5–25.0	25.5–30.0	30.5+
50+	16	16.5–21.5	22.0–26.0	26.5–31.0	31.5+
Women					
<19	17	17.5–22.0	22.5–27.0	27.5–32.0	32.5+
20–29	18	18.5–23.0	23.5–28.0	28.5–33.0	33.5+
30–39	19	19.5–24.0	24.5–29.0	29.5–34.0	34.5+
40–49	20	20.5–25.0	25.5–30.0	30.5–35.0	35.5+
50+	21	21.5–26.5	27.0–31.0	31.5–36.0	36.5+

*Round percent fat to nearest 0.5%. Ideal classification is based on health-related fitness, not athletic performance per se.
Source: Hoeger (1989).

BODY COMPOSITION

inversely related to percent body fat. In other words, as body density increases, percent fat decreases.

Body density is defined as *mass-per-unit volume*. In the measurement of body density, mass can be easily measured with a standard weight scale. Body volume, on the other hand, is more difficult to measure because it requires utilization of Archimedes' principle of water displacement. (Please review reference material for additional information on body volume measurement.)

A simple way to conceptualize hydrostatic weighing is to realize that fat floats in water and lean mass (muscle, bone, etc.) sinks. If a person sinks easily in water, he or she probably has a high proportion of lean weight versus fat weight. Conversely, if a person floats in water following a complete exhalation, a high percentage of fat throughout the body is probable.

Although hydrostatic weighing is the standard test for body composition analysis, it too only estimates actual levels of body fat. The only way to obtain an exact measurement of body fat is to excise and measure all the fat from a cadaver. Since hydrostatic weighing is a valid non-invasive means of assessing body composition, exercise scientists continue to use it as the standard method of body composition assessment. Most other methods of body composition assessment (i.e., skinfold measures, electrical impedance, etc.) are validated in reference to hydrostatic weighing results.

In most circumstances, hydrostatic weighing is the preferred method for body composition analysis; however, several factors limit its general use. For instance, the test requires trained administrators and special equipment; it takes time and may be somewhat inconvenient to perform; and certain people have a difficult time performing the test because of hydrophobia or the inability to exhale completely.

Because hydrostatic weighing is the standard method of body composition assessment, a new method is validated according to its ability to predict hydrostatic weighing results. (See Chapter 1.) For example, the $\sum 3$ and $\sum 7$ skinfold methods used in this lab have correlations to hydrostatic weighing of 0.85–0.90. The SEE for skinfolds is approximately 3–4% BF depending on the calipers used, obesity of the subject, and the experience of the administrator.

SELECTED REFERENCES

Adams, G. M. (1990). *Exercise Physiology Lab Manual*. Dubuque Iowa: Wm. C. Brown Publishers, pp: 187–225.

American College of Sports Medicine (1991). *Guidelines of Exercise Testing and Prescription* (4th edition). Philadelphia: Lea & Febiger, pp: 43–48.

Behnke, A.R., and J. H. Wilmore (1974). *Evaluation and Regulation of Body Build and Composition*. Englewood Cliffs, New Jersey: Prentice Hall.

Brozek, J., F. Grande, J. Anderson, and A. Keys (1963). Densitometric analysis of body composition: revision of some quantitative assumptions. *Annals of the New York Academy of Sciences* 110:113–140.

DeVries, H. A. (1986). *Physiology of Exercise: For Physical Education and Athletics* (4th edition). Dubuque, Iowa: Wm. C. Brown Publishers, pp: 338–344.

DiGirolamo, M. (1986, March). Body composition—roundtable. *The Physician and Sportsmedicine* 14: 144–162.

Fisher, A. G., and C. R. Jensen (1990). *Scientific Basis of Athletic Conditioning* (3rd edition). Philadelphia: Lea & Febiger, pp: 257–259.

Fitness and Amateur Sport Canada (1986). *Canadian Standardized Test of Fitness* (3rd edition). Ottawa.

Fox, E. L., R. W. Bowers, and M. L. Foss (1988). *The Physiological Basis of Physical Education and Athletics* (4th edition). Philadelphia: Saunders College Publishing, pp: 564–570.

Goldman, H. L. and M. R. Becklace (1959). Respiratory function tests: normal values of medium altitude and the prediction of normal results. *Am. Rev. Tuber. Respir. Dis.* 79: 457–469.

Heyward, V. H. (1991). *Advanced Fitness Assessment and Exercise Prescription*. Champaign, Illinois: Human Kinetics, pp: 17–69.

Hoeger, W. W. K. (1989). *Lifetime Physical Fitness and Wellness: A Personalized Program*. Englewood, Colorado: Morton Publishing Company, pp: 101–115.

Howley, E. T., and D. B. Frank (1992). *Health Fitness Instructor's Handbook* (2nd edition). Champaign, Illinois: Human Kinetics, pp: 116–125.

Jackson, A. S., and M. L. Pollock (1978). Generalized equations for predicting body density of men. *British Journal of Nutrition* 40: 497–504.

Katch, F. I., T. Hortobagyi, and T. Denahan (1989). Reliability and validity of a new method for the measurement of total body volume. *Research Quarterly for Exercise and Sport* 60(3):286–291.

Keys, A., F. Fidanza, M. J. Karvonen, N. Kimura, and H. L. Taylor (1972). Relative merits of the weight-corrected-for-height indices. *The American Journal of Clinical Nutrition* 34:2521–2529.

Lohman, T.G. (1981). Skinfolds and body density and their relation to body fatness: a review. *Hum Biology* 53(2):181–225.

Lamb, D. R. (1984). *Physiology of Exercise: Responses and Adaptations* (2nd edition). New York: Macmillan Publishing Company, pp: 114–121.

McArdle, W. D., F. I. Katch, and V. L. Katch (1991). *Exercise Physiology: Energy, Nutrition, and Human Performance* (3rd edition). Philadelphia: Lea & Febiger, pp: 599–633.

Noble, B. J. (1986). *Physiology of Exercise and Sport*. St.Louis, Missouri: Times Mirror/Mosby College Publishing, pp: 325–333, 349–355.

Penrose K. W., A. G. Nelson, and A. G. Fisher (1985). *Generalized Body Composition Prediction Equation for Men Using Simple Measurement Techniques.* Unpublished doctoral dissertation.

Pollock M. L., J. H. Wilmore, and S. M. Fox (1990). *Exercise in Health and Disease, Evaluation and Prescription for Prevention and Rehabilitation.* Philadelphia: Saunders College Publishing.

Powers, S. K., and E. T. Howley (1990). *Exercise Physiology: Theory and Application to Fitness and Performance.* Dubuque, Iowa: Wm. C. Brown Publishers, pp: 381–389.

Siri, W. E. (1961). Body composition from fluid spaces and density: analysis of methods. In: Brozek, J., and Henshel, A. eds, *Techniques for Measuring Body Composition.* Washington, DC: National Academy of Sciences-National Research Council, pp: 223–244.

Vehrs, P. R., J. D. George, C. Payne, J. Peugnet, G. R. Bryce, G. W. Fellingham, and A. G. Fisher (1993). Reliability of near-infrared interactance, electrical impedance, and bottle buoyancy in determining body composition. *Medicine and Science in Sport and Exercise* 25(5):5, Abstract #29.

Wilmore, J. H., and D. L. Costill (1988). *Training for Sport and Activity: The Physiological Basis of the Conditioning Process* (3rd edition). Dubuque, Iowa: Wm. C. Brown Publishers, pp: 375–384.

STATION 1
. . . .
Body Composition Prediction Methods

Research Questions

1. How does your BMI compare to your waist-to-hip ratio? Is there any logical relationship between these two measures? Do you think it is possible that someone might have a normal BMI, yet have a high waist-to-hip ratio? Which test do you see as most valuable when measuring health-related physical fitness? Explain.

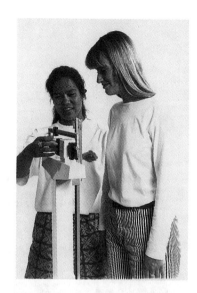

2. If the department of Physical Education/Exercise Science required all graduating majors to have a percent body fat not higher than 15% for males and 22% for females, would you meet this graduation requirement using the height-squared index, circumference measures, and skinfold measures? In your answer provide a summary of your results. Do you think this is a reasonable requirement? Why and why not? Do you think it is fair to establish similar body composition guidelines as a criteria for enlistment in the armed services? Justify your response.

3. Compare the results of the $\sum 3$ and $\sum 7$ skinfold measurements. Do they predict similar body densities? Do they predict similar percent body fat values? Should they? Why or why not? What are some of the sources of error of the skinfold technique?

Data Collection

1. With a partner, perform each of the prediction tests described below.
2. Record your results on the appropriate data sheet.

Body Mass Index (BMI)
The BMI is a simple weight-to-height ratio. The theory behind this method is that weight-to-height ratios across the general population have a positive relationship with percent body fat. BMI is commonly used as an indicator of obesity and is correlated to an increased risk of cardiovascular disease.

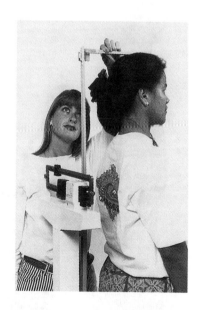

1. Measure your body weight (kg) and height (m).
2. Calculate your BMI based on the formula below.

$$\text{BMI} = \text{Body Weight (kg)} \div \text{Height}^2 \text{ (meters)}$$

3. Record your results in Chart 6–1.

Computation Example: What is the BMI of a 76-inch-tall male weighing 187 pounds? Identify the obesity category using the BMI.

1. Convert his body height to meters and body weight to kg.

$$76 \text{ inches} \times \frac{2.54 \text{ cm}}{\text{inch}} = 193.0 \text{ cm} \times \frac{1 \text{ meter}}{100 \text{ cm}} = 1.93 \text{ m}$$

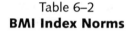

$$187 \text{ lbs} \times \frac{0.4536 \text{ kg}}{\text{pound}} = 84.8 \text{ kg}$$

2. Compute his BMI. Even though the unit values for the BMI would be kg/m², the index is generally reported with no unit values.

$$\text{BMI} = \text{Wt} \div \text{Ht}^2 = 84.8 \text{ kg} \div 1.93^2 = 22.76$$

3. Obesity Category = Non-Obese.

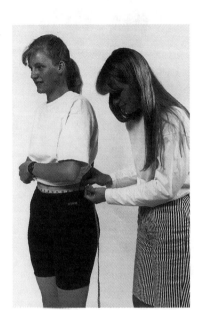

Table 6–2
BMI Index Norms

Classification	Men	Women
Non-obese	<25	<27
Moderately obese	25–30	27–30
Obese	>30	>30

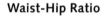

Source: Adapted from DiGirolamo (1986).

Waist-Hip Ratio

The waist-hip (W/H) ratio is an index used to estimate the risk of cardiovascular disease associated with obesity. A high ratio (i.e., relatively high amounts of fat located in the abdominal area) has been found to pose a greater risk of cardiovascular disease than a low ratio.

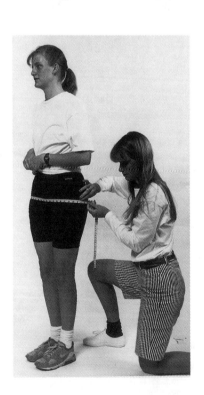

1. Have your partner measure your waist or abdominal circumference at the smallest circumference below the rib cage and above the umbilicus.
2. With your feet together, have your partner measure your hip or gluteal circumference at the largest circumference (greatest posterior protrusion) of the buttocks.
3. Calculate your ratio by dividing your waist measurement by your hip measurement. Make sure you use the same unit values (inches or centimeters) for each measurement.
4. Record your results in Chart 6–1.

Computation Example: What is the W/H ratio of a 25-yr-old female who has a waist measurement of 32 inches and a hip measurement of 42 inches? What is her waist-to-hip percentile norm rating and does her measurement fall within an estimated health risk zone (Table 6–3)?

1. $\text{W} / \text{H} = \dfrac{\text{Waist Measurement}}{\text{Hip Measurement}} = \dfrac{32 \text{ inches}}{42 \text{ inches}} = 0.76$

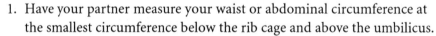

2. Percentile norm rating: 40th percentile; No.

Table 6–3
Waist-to-Hip Ratio Norms*
(Abdominal to Gluteal Ratio Norms)

	15–19 yr		20–29 yr		30–39 yr		40–49 yr		50–59 yr		60–69 yr	
Pctl	M	F	M	F	M	F	M	F	M	F	M	F
95	.73	.65	.76	.65	.80	.66	.81	.66	.82	.67	.84	.71
90	.75	.67	.80	.67	.81	.68	.83	.69	.85	.71	.88	.73
85	.76	.68	.81	.68	.82	.69	.84	.71	.87	.72	.89	.74
80	.77	.69	.81	.69	.83	.71	.86	.72	.89	.73	.90	.75
75	.79	.71	.82	.71	.84	.72	.87	.73	.89	.74	.90	.76
70	.80	.72	.83	.72	.84	.73	.88	.74	.90	.75	.91.	77
65	.81	.73	.83	.73	.85	.74	.89	.75	.91	.76	.92	.78
60	.81	.73	.84	.73	.86	.75	.90	.76	.92	.77	.93	.79
55	.82	.74	.85	.74	.87	.75	.91	.76	.92	.77	.94	.80
50	.83	.75	.85	.75	.88	.76	.92	.77	.93	.78	.94	.81
45	.83	.75	.86	.76	.89	.77	.92	.78	.94	.79	.95	.82
40	.84	.76	.87	.76	.90	.78	.93	.79	.95	.80	.96	.83
35	.85	.77	.87	.77	.91	.78	.94	.79	.95	.81	.97	.84
30	.85	.78	.88	.78	.92	.79	.95	.80	.96	.82	.98	.85
25	.86	.78	.89	.78	.93	.80	.95	.82	.98	.84	.99	.86
20	.87	.79	.91	.79	.94	.81	.97	.84	.99	.85	1.00	.87
15	.87	.80	.93	.80	.95	.83	.99	.86	1.01	.86	1.02	.88
10	.88	.82	.94	.82	.96	.85	1.01	.87	1.02	.88	1.03	.91
5	.92	.86	.96	.85	1.01	.87	1.03	.92	1.04	.92	1.04	.94

*Percentile and associated health risk zones by age groups and gender.

☐ = Estimated health risk zones based on trends in morbidity and mortality data.

Source: Adapted from the *Canadian Standardized Test of Fitness (CSTF) Operations Manual* (3rd edition), 1986. Used with permission from the Canadian Society for Exercise Physiology in cooperation with the Government of Canada.

Height-Squared Index

The Height-Squared Index is based on a simple regression formula (Behnke and Wilmore, 1974) that estimates lean body mass (LBM) based on body height. The underlying theory behind this test is that body height, over the general population, has a positive relationship with lean body weight.

1. Remove your shoes and measure your height to the nearest 1/4 inch. Also measure your body weight to the nearest 1/4 pound.
2. Convert height to decimeters (1 inch = 2.54 cm = 0.254 dm) and convert pounds to kilograms (1 pound = 0.4536 kg).
3. Use the appropriate regression equation to compute LBM

Men: LBM (kg) = 0.204 x Ht^2 (height in decimeters)
Women: LBM (kg) = 0.18 x Ht^2 (height in decimeters)

BODY COMPOSITION
113

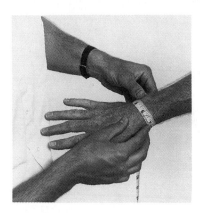

4. Percent fat = $\dfrac{\text{Body weight (kg)} - \text{LBM (kg)}}{\text{Body Weight (kg)}} \times 100$

5. Record your results in Chart 6-1.

Computation Example: What is the height-squared index of a 21-year-old male who is 72 inches tall? What would be his %BF if he weighed 95 kg?

$$\text{LBM (kg)} = 0.204 \times (72 \text{ inches} \times 0.254 \text{ dm/inch})^2 = 68.22 \text{ kg}$$

$$\%\text{BF} = \dfrac{95 \text{ kg} - 68.228 \text{ kg}}{95 \text{ kg}} \times 100 = 28.18\% \text{ BF}$$

Girth/Circumference Measurements

The measurement of circumferences (girths) of specific body parts can be used to predict %BF since it is assumed that these measures have a positive relationship to percent body fat. Thus, as body girths increase, it is assumed that body fat levels also increase.

1. Have a partner measure the circumferences listed below. Use a cloth tape measure and pull the tape lightly but firmly around the areas to be measured. Be sure to keep the tape level during the measurement and if possible to measure over bare skin. Take two or three measurements at each measurement site and record the average score on Chart 6–1.

   Male Circumference Sites:
   Wrist (WR): Measure around the wrist just distal to the radial and ulnar styloid processes.
   Abdomen (AC): Measure around the abdomen at the level of the umbilicus.

   Female Circumference Sites:
   Abdomen (AC): Measure around the abdomen at the level of the umbilicus.
   Hip (HC): Measure around the hips or buttocks at the maximum girth. Have your subject stand with feet together.

2. Compute your predicted %BF with the appropriate gender-specific regression equation below. Note that each equation is designed for college-aged individuals.

   Male (Penrose, Nelson, and Fisher, 1985):

   $$\text{LBM (kg)} = 41.955 + (1.03876 \times \text{WT}) - (0.82816 \times (\text{AC} - \text{WR}))^*$$

   $$\%\text{BF} = \dfrac{\text{Body Weight} - \text{Lean Body Weight}}{\text{Body Weight}}$$

   Female:

   $$\%\text{BF} = (0.55 \times \text{HC}) - (0.24 \times \text{Ht}) + (0.28 \times \text{AC}) - 8.43^\dagger$$

Where: WT = Body weight; (kg)

　　　AC = Abdominal circumference (level with umbilicus); (cm)

　　　WR = Wrist circumference; (cm)

　　　HC = Hip circumference (cm)

　　　Ht = Body height; (cm)

*Courtesy of Richard W. Coté and Jack H. Wilmore

3. Record your results in Chart 6–1.

Computation Example: A 25 year-old-female is 65 inches tall, has an abdominal circumference of 70 cm, and a hip circumference of 90 cm. What is her predicted percent body fat?

1. Convert her height from inches to centimeters.

$$65 \text{ inches} \times \frac{2.54 \text{ cm}}{1 \text{ inch}} = 165.1 \text{ cm}$$

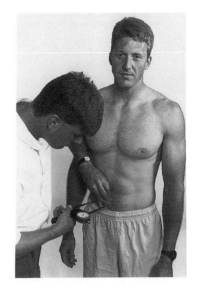

2. Compute her %BF using the circumference regression equation

%BF = (0.55 × HC) − (0.24 × Ht) + (0.28 × AC) − 8.43

%BF = (0.55 × 90) − (0.24 × 165.1) + (0.28 × 70) − 8.43

%BF = 21%

Rating = Good

Skinfold Measurements

The measurement of subcutaneous skinfolds is used to predict body density or percent body fat. It is assumed that subcutaneous fat has a positive relationship with total body fat (i.e., as subcutaneous body fat increases, total body fat increases). The sum of several skinfolds is used to predict %BF or body density as determined by hydrostatic weighing. Body fat results are usually obtained using regression equations or nomograms.

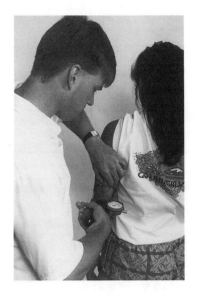

1. Have a partner measure the appropriate skinfold measurements at the landmark sites listed below. Note in the calculation that males and females have gender-specific measurement sites.

> *Skinfold Technique*: Measure the thickness of a skinfold on the *right* side of the body. Firmly pinch the skin and subcutaneous fat between the thumb and index finger. Open the caliper and measure the skinfold approximately 1 cm below your fingers and approximately 1 cm deep into the skinfold. Do not release the skinfold from between your fingers while the caliper is attached to it. Be sure to pinch all of the fat. You may wish to request your subject to flex the muscle under the skinfold to make it easier for you to pinch the subcutaneous fat. Note that your skinfold should follow the natural cleavage of the skin and will normally be parallel to the muscle immediately below your measurement site (i.e., the triceps muscle and triceps skinfold are parallel to one another).

Take three measurements, at least 15 seconds apart, at each skinfold site. You may wish to perform your skinfold measurements in a circuit, that is, rotate from one site to another to allow for the 15-second time interval between individual site measurements. The gauge of the caliper should be read to the closest half millimeter (e.g., Lange) or tenth millimeter (e.g., Harpenden). Record the average of the three skinfold measurements on Chart 6–2.

Landmark Skinfold Measurement Sites

Chest: A diagonal fold taken one half of the distance between the anterior axillary line and the nipple

Axilla: A vertical fold on the mid-axillary line at the level of the xiphoid process of the sternum.

Triceps: A vertical fold on the posterior midline of the upper arm, halfway between the acromion and olecranon processes.

Subscapula: A diagonal fold from the vertebral border to 1–2 cm below the scapular inferior angle.

Abdominal: A vertical fold taken at a lateral distance of approximately 2 cm from the umbilicus.

Suprailium: A diagonal fold above the crest of the ilium at the spot where an imaginary line would be drawn from the anterior axillary line.

Thigh: A vertical fold on the anterior aspect of the thigh, halfway between the midpoint of the inguinal ligament and the proximal border of the patella. Note: The midpoint of the inguinal ligament is halfway between the anterior superior iliac spine and the symphysis pubis.

2. The sum of three ($\sum 3$) and seven ($\sum 7$) skinfolds is frequently used to predict body density. Calculate body density (Db) with the appropriate $\sum 3$ and $\sum 7$ skinfold equations (Pollock, Wilmore, and Fox, 1990) listed below:

Males:

$$Db\ (\textstyle\sum 3) = 1.10938 - (0.0008267 \times \textstyle\sum 3) + (0.0000016 \times \textstyle\sum 3^2) - (0.0002574 \times age)$$

$$Db\ (\textstyle\sum 7) = 1.1120 - (0.00043499 \times \textstyle\sum 7) + (0.00000055 \times \textstyle\sum 7^2) - (0.00028826 \times age)$$

Females:

$$Db\ (\textstyle\sum 3) = 1.0994921 - (0.0009929 \times \textstyle\sum 3) + (0.0000023 \times \textstyle\sum 3^2) - (0.0001392 \times age)$$

$$Db\ (\textstyle\sum 7) = 1.0970 - (0.00046971 \times \textstyle\sum 7) + (0.00000056 \times \textstyle\sum 7^2) - (0.00012828 \times age)$$

Db = Body density

$\sum 3$ = Sum of chest, abdomen, and thigh skinfolds (mm) for males

$\sum 3$ = Sum of triceps, suprailium, and thigh skinfolds (mm) for females

$\sum 7$ = Sum of chest, axilla, triceps, subscapula, abdominal, supraillium, and thigh skinfolds (mm) for both males and females.

3. Calculate %BF from Siri's following body density equation (Siri, 1961):

$$\%BF = ((4.95/Db) - 4.50) \times 100$$

4. Record your results on Chart 6–3.

Computation Example: A 22-year-old female is measured to have $\sum 3$ skinfolds of 55 mm and $\sum 7$ skinfolds of 105 mm. What is her estimated body density and percent body fat?

$$Db\ (\textstyle\sum 3) = 1.0994921 - (0.0009929 \times 55) + (0.0000023 \times 55^2) - (0.0001392 \times 22) =$$

$$Db\ (\textstyle\sum 3) = 1.0994921 - (0.0546) + (0.0000023 \times 3025) - (0.003062) =$$

$$Db\ (\textstyle\sum 3) = 1.0994921 - (0.0546) + (0.00695) - (0.003062) = 1.04878$$
or 1.0488

$$\%BF = ((4.95/1.0488) - 4.50) \times 100 =$$

$$\%BF = (4.7196 - 4.50) \times 100 =$$

$$\%BF = (0.2196) \times 100 = 21.97 \text{ or } 22.0$$

$$Db\ (\textstyle\sum 7) = 1.0970 - (0.00046971 \times 105) + (0.00000056 \times 105^2) - (0.00012828 \times 22) =$$

$$Db\ (\textstyle\sum 7) = 1.0970 - (0.049318) + (0.00000056 \times 11025) - (0.0028204) =$$

$$Db\ (\textstyle\sum 7) = 1.0970 - (0.0493) + (0.0062) - (0.0028) = 1.0511$$
or 1.0504

$$\%BF = ((4.95/1.0511) - 4.50) \times 100 =$$

$$\%BF = (4.7094 - 4.50) \times 100 =$$

$$\%BF = (0.2094) \times 100 = 20.94$$

Answers:

	Σ3 Skinfolds	Σ7 Skinfolds
Predicted Db	1.0488	1.0504
%BF	22.0	20.9
Rating	Good	Good

Wrist - 17.5cm 15

Belly - 74cm 78

Waist - 77cm 78 99

Hip - 102cm

136.4   31.5
        27.5

STATION 2
Hydrostatic Weighing

This station is optional depending on the availability of hydrostatic weighing equipment in your laboratory.

Research Questions

1. Do the results appear realistic? (Does it seem logical that the person evaluated would have this percent fat? Explain.)

2. If the person evaluated actually has an RV 500 ml higher than utilized, would this increase or decrease the body fat composition? What would be the measurement error? Discuss implications.

3. Describe how the subject, administrator, and equipment each could increase the measurement error of hydrostatic weighing. Provide specific examples.

4. Explain why hydrostatic weighing as the standard method is more accurate than skinfold and circumference measurements (prediction methods), assuming all test protocols are properly performed.

5. Discuss the various advantages and disadvantages of the traditional hydrostatic method. Discuss the various advantages and disadvantages of the Natant hydrostatic method.

Data Collection

A volunteer from the lab will perform the traditional and/or Natant hydrostatic weighing procedures. Your lab instructor will provide you with the appropriate body density and percent fat data. In the event your laboratory is not equipped to do this test, your instructor may provide the required data.

Traditional Hydrostatic Weighing
1. Compute the percent fat of your volunteer based on the data provided by your instructor. Show your work.
2. Record your test results in Charts 6–4 and 6–5.

   Total body volume (TBV) and body density (Db) are calculated with the equations below. Percent body fat is calculated from density (Db) with the Siri (1962) equation.

$$TBV = \frac{(Ma - Mw)}{Dw} - (RV + VGI)$$

$$Db = Ma \div TBV$$

$$\%BF = ((4.95/Db) - 4.50) \times 100$$

Where: Ma = body mass in air (kg)

Mw = body mass in water

Dw = temperature correction for water density

RV = residual volume (liters, estimated or measured and corrected to BTPS)*

VGI = volume of gas in the gastrointestinal tract (equals about 100 ml or 0.1 liters)

* If measurement of residual volume is not possible, RV can be estimated with the following equations (Goldman and Becklace, 1959). A discussion about the BTPS correction factor is located in Chapter 13.

Males:

$$RV_{BTPS} (L) = (0.017 \times age) + (0.06858 \times height; inches) - 3.477$$

Females:

$$RV_{BTPS} (L) = (0.009 \times age) + (0.08128 \times height; inches) - 3.90$$

Record data and compute results on Chart 6-4.

Computation Example: What are the hydrostatic weighing results for a 25-year-old male subject based on the following data: Mass in air (Ma) = 80.5 kg; mass in water (Mw) = 3.5 kg; residual volume = 1.9 L; water temperature = 35°C; and intestinal gas (VGI) = 0.1 L. Compute percent fat with the Siri formula.

The percent fat for a 25-year-old male subject using traditional hydrostatic weighing would be:

$$TBV = \frac{(Ma - Mw)}{Dw} - (RV + VGL)$$

$$TBV = \frac{80.5 \text{ kg} - 3.5 \text{ kg}}{0.994063} \ (1.9 \text{ L} + 0.1 \text{L}) = 75.45 \text{ L}$$

$$Dw = 0.994063$$

Body density (Db) = Ma ÷ TBV

Db = 80.5 kg ÷ 75.45 L = 1.0669 or 1.067

Percent body fat (Siri) = [(4.95/Db) – 4.50] × 100

%BF = ((4.95/1.0669) – 4.50) × 100 = 13.9%

Be sure to express body density (Db) to at least four decimal places (i.e., 0.9945 and not 0.99), otherwise you will not compute accurate % fat scores.

Natant Hydrostatic Weighing

1. Your instructor will demonstrate the Natant procedure and provide you with all necessary data.
2. Record the test results in Chart 6–5.

Recent research has demonstrated that Natant is a valid and reliable measurement of body density and percent fat. The reliability and validity coefficients of Natant have been shown to be 0.99 when compared to traditional hydrostatic weighing. For further information regarding the Natant system please refer to McArdle, Katch, and Katch, 1991, pp. 612-615; Katch, Hortobagyi, and Denahan, 1989; and Vehrs et al.,1993.

Note: The authors can send you further information on how to acquire the Natant hydrostatic weighing system. Address correspondence to Jim George. (See Appendix E.)

Table 6–4
Temperature Corrections for Water Density

Water Temp	Dw	Water Temp	Dw
23°C	0.997569	30°C	0.995678
24°C	0.997327	31°C	0.995372
25°C	0.997075	32°C	0.995057
26°C	0.996814	33°C	0.994734
27°C	0.996544	34°C	0.994403
28°C	0.996264	35°C	0.994063
29°C	0.995976	36°C	0.993716

2.33
29°C

Water
3.6
3.65
3.7
3.7
3.65

1.37

. . . .
Lab 6 Summary

How can the information learned from this lab be applied to your specific field of interest and/or your personal life. Be specific and provide practical examples.

Name: _____   Date: _____

7

Assessment of Overall Physical Fitness
· ·
Pre-Laboratory Assignment

1. What is your personal definition of physical fitness? Be specific and elaborate.

2. What is the difference between norm-reference standards and criterion-reference standards? Provide an example of each.

3. What is the estimated VO_{2max} ($ml \cdot kg^{-1} \cdot min^{-1}$) of a college female who is 22 years old, has a body weight of 140 lbs, and ran the 1.5 mile run in 14:33 min:sec? Show your work.

4. ☐ Check the box if you have read each research question for this lab and are familiar with the data collection procedures regarding each research question.

7

Assessment of Overall Physical Fitness

PURPOSE
The purpose of this lab is to provide additional practice measuring the five health-related components of physical fitness.

STUDENT LEARNING OBJECTIVES
1. Be able to administer a comprehensive physical fitness evaluation.
2. Be able to describe how each component of physical fitness influences overall physical fitness.

NECESSARY EQUIPMENT
Stop watch
Stethoscope and sphygmomanometer
Weight-lifting equipment
Sit-and-reach board
Cardiorespiratory endurance test equipment
Natant hydrostatic weighing system
Skin fold calipers
Measuring tape
Weight scale

FITNESS ASSESSMENT
An overall physical fitness assessment is very common in health clubs, recreation centers, schools, and corporations. As noted in prior labs, physical fitness testing is valuable in that individual strengths and weaknesses can be evaluated; safe, effective training programs can be designed; realistic goals can be established; progress can be tracked; and motivation can possibly be enhanced. Fitness assessments are also used by corporations as screening tools to determine if employees are capable of performing required work tasks with minimal risk of injury. Related types of testing are also valuable in determining if and when employees are able to return to work following an injury.

All five components of physical fitness should be measured when overall physical fitness is evaluated. Fitness assessments should be administered in a standardized manner to ensure validity and reliability. The type of test employed to assess physical fitness depends on the purpose(s) of the test, the degree of accuracy required, the expense, the availability of trained personnel, and the necessary equipment.

Test results for a given physical fitness evaluation can be rated based on norm-reference standards or criterion-reference standards. Normative ratings, as discussed in Chapter 1, are simply a percentile ranking (i.e., above 85th percentile = excellent category) that indicate how one compares with others of the same gender and similar age. Criterion-reference ratings, on the other hand, reflect whether or not a certain level of fitness, often associated with such things as good health or optimal job performance, have been met. The Physical Best program developed by AAHPERD suggests certain health-related criterion standards. The United States Air Force ROTC program (AFROTC) along with many other vocations (e.g., police, fire services) have established specific performance-related criterion standards.

Outlined below are potential advantages and disadvantages of both norm-reference and criterion-reference standards.

Norm-Reference Standards

Advantages:

a. Ratings are relatively easy to compute, since it is a simple percentile ranking system.

b. They provide objective means to compare oneself to others of similar age and the same gender.

Disadvantages:

a. Normative data do not always correlate with good health or reduced risk of disease. Thus a high rating doesn't always equate to good health; conversely a low rating doesn't always imply poor health.

b. A high rating may not be achievable by many individuals in a given population because of genetic limitations, regardless of their physical activity and/or dietary habits.

c. An individual who earns a low rating even though physically active may experience decreased motivation for continued participation.

Criterion-Reference Standards

Advantages:

a. Ratings are explicitly linked to a criterion score that is associated with a given health or performance status.

b. They represent an absolute minimal level that may be consistent with optimal health or performance. Because criterion-reference standards are absolute, it is possible that either a very high or a very low proportion of the population may meet a desired standard.

c. An individual who fails to pass a given criterion-reference standard immediately knows whether lifestyle habits—physical activity and/or dietary—should be modified.

Disadvantages:

a. Cut-off scores may be arbitrary. This problem is more common with health-related standards since it is difficult to know the exact minimal level that is associated with good health. Performance-related standards are less arbitrary, however, since specific physical job requirements (e.g., fire fighting) can be ascertained and minimal fitness levels established.

b. There may be misclassifications. Some may be misclassified and have the false impression they are healthy and/or competent, when in actuality they are not. Conversely, some may be falsely classified as unfit and consequently view themselves as unhealthy and/or incompetent.

c. Criterion-reference standards for health-related fitness tests represent desired minimum levels of fitness and therefore may not provide sufficient incentive for some individuals to achieve increased levels of fitness. On the other hand, individuals who fail to pass the health-related standard even though they are physically active may have a decreased motivation for continued participation.

SELECTED REFERENCES

AAHPERD (1988). *The AAHPERD Physical Best Program.* Reston, Virginia: American Alliance for Health, Physical Education, Recreation, and Dance.

Air Force ROTC (1992). AFROTCR 35–2, Attachment 7.

American College of Sports Medicine (1988). Opinion statement on physical fitness in children and youth. *Medicine and Science in Sports and Exercise,* 20:422–423.

American College of Sports Medicine (1988). *Guidelines for Exercise Testing and Prescription Resource Manual.* Institute for Aerobics Research, pp:161–170.

American College of Sports Medicine (1990). Position stand on the recommended quantity and quality of exercise for developing and maintaining cardiorespiratory and muscular fitness in healthy adults. *Medicine and Science in Sports and Exercise,* 22:265–274.

American Heart Association (1992). Statement on exercise. *Circulation,* 86(1):2726–2730.

Cureton, K. J., and G. L. Warren (1990). Criterion-referenced standards for youth health-related fitness tests: a tutorial. *Research Quarterly for Exercise and Sport,* 61(1):7–19.

George, J. D., P. R. Vehrs, P. E. Allsen, G. W. Fellingham, and A. G. Fisher (1993). VO_{2max} estimation from a submaximal 1-mile track jog for fit college-age individuals. *Medicine and Science in Sports and Exercise,* 25(3):401–406.

George, J. D., P. R. Vehrs, P. E. Allsen, G. W. Fellingham, and A. G. Fisher (1993). Development of a submaximal treadmill jogging test for fit college-aged individuals. *Medicine and Science in Sports and Exercise,* 25(5):643–647.

Golding, L. A., C. R. Myers, and W. E. Sinning (Eds.) (1989). *The Y's Way to Physical Fitness,* 3rd edition. Champaign, Illinois: Human Kinetics Books.

Pate, R. R. (1988). The evolving definition of physical fitness. *Quest,* 40:174–179.

STATION 1
. . . .
Assessment of Physical Fitness

Research Questions

1. Based on norm-reference standards, are you above average on the applicable physical fitness tests assigned by your instructor? Estimate what percent of your current level of fitness is attributed to your genetic endowment, exercise habits, and nutritional habits, respectively. Explain.

2. Based on AAHPERD health-related criterion-reference standards (18-year-old standards), do you satisfy the minimum score on the applicable physical fitness tests assigned by your instructor? Do you feel you possess a level of physical fitness that is associated with good health? Explain.

3. Based on AFROTC performance-related criterion-reference standards, do you satisfy the minimum score on the applicable physical fitness tests assigned by your instructor? Do you think the military should use health-related standards or performance-related standards to rate their applicants? Justify your answer.

4. With regard to overall physical fitness, what are your strengths and weaknesses? Are you content with your overall level of physical fitness?

5. Why would it be an advantage to improve and/or maintain your current level of physical fitness?

6. Outline several ways you could change your current lifestyle (exercise, nutritional habits, etc.) to improve your physical fitness. Be specific.

Data Collection

If you have successfully completed the first six chapters of this laboratory text, you should have the skills necessary to measure the overall physical fitness of apparently healthy individuals of any age. Your instructor should inform you of which physical fitness tests you are to perform. Note that you may be assigned to practice tests already performed in previous chapters and/or be assigned to conduct tests presented in this chapter.

Work with a partner and assist one another in evaluating each test item assigned. Refer to information in this lab and/or previous labs for specific data collection procedures, normative-reference standards, and criterion-reference standards. Remember that the purpose of this lab is to provide you with further practice and experience measuring the various components of physical fitness.

Comprehensive Physical Fitness Evaluation

Resting heart rate and blood pressure
1. Palpate your partner's radial pulse for 1 minute. Record the results (see Chapter 7 assignment).
2. Measure your partner's resting blood pressure using a stethoscope and a sphygmomanometer. Repeat this measurement at least twice to ensure that the blood pressure you record is correct.

Astrand Cycle Test
Rockport Walking Test
George-Fisher Jogging Test
Forest Service Step Test
1. Instructions and norms for these tests are found in Chapter 5.
2. Record your test results and normative rating(s) on Chart 7–1 on page 153.

Treadmill jogging test
1. If available, secure an electronic heart rate monitor around the chest of your partner. (Be sure there is moisture under the chest contact points.) Attach the wristwatch receiver to the front or side railing of the treadmill within 2–3 ft of your subject.
2. Warm up your partner at a brisk treadmill walking speed (3.5–4.5 mph).
3. Have your partner self-select a comfortable jogging speed that is $\leq$ 6.5 mph for females and $\leq$ 7.5 mph for males.
4. Allow your partner to jog at a steady pace for at least 3 minutes until a steady-state heart rate is achieved. (Exercise heart rate is considered at steady-state when consecutive HRs (30 seconds apart) differ by $\leq$ 3 bpm after about 3 minutes of jogging.) Note that the test is invalid if exercise HRs exceed 180 bpm. In the event you don't have an electronic heart rate monitor, have your partner momentarily straddle the treadmill belt and immediately palpate a 10-second pulse count.
5. Record the steady-state heart rate (bpm) of your partner. Slow the treadmill speed and allow your subject to walk (cool down) for several minutes.
6. Based on your own data, use the accompanying regression equation to compute VO_{2max}.
7. Record your test results and normative rating on Chart 7–1.

Treadmill jogging test regression equation*

$$VO_{2max} \text{ (ml}^{-1}\cdot\text{kg}^{-1}\cdot\text{min}^{-1}) = 54.07 + (7.062 \times G) - (0.1938 \times BW)$$
$$+ (4.47 \times S) - (0.1453 \times HR)$$

Where:
    G = Gender (0 = female; 1 = male)
    BW = Body weight (kg)
    S = Speed of treadmill (mph)
    HR = Steady-state exercise heart rate (bpm)

*Source: George et al. (May 1993)

Computation example: What is the estimated VO_{2max} ($ml·kg^{-1}·min^{-1}$) of a college female who is 19 years old, has a body weight of 155 lbs, a treadmill jogging speed of 5.7 mph, and an exercise heart rate of 171 bpm? Show your work.

1.   Convert body weight from pounds to kilograms:

$$155\,lbs \times \frac{1\,kg}{2.2\,lbs} = 70.45\,kg$$

2. Compute an estimate of VO_{2max} with the following regression equation:

$$VO_{2max}\ (ml·kg^{-1}·min^{-1}) = 54.07 + (7.062 \times G)$$
$$- (0.1938 \times BW) + (4.47 \times S) - (0.1453 \times HR)$$

$$VO_{2max}\ (ml·kg^{-1}·min^{-1}) = 54.07 + (7.062 \times 0) - (0.1938 \times 70.45)$$
$$+ (4.47 \times 5.7) - (0.1453 \times 171)$$

$$VO_{2max}\ (ml·kg^{-1}·min^{-1}) = 54.07 + (13.65) + (25.47) - (24.84)$$

$$VO_{2max} = 41.05\ ml·kg^{-1}·min^{-1}$$

Fitness Level: Good (See Table 5–1).

1.5 mile run

1. Run 1.5 miles as fast as possible over a level surface (i.e., track). Have your partner record your time. Be sure to pace yourself during the run to help prevent premature fatigue.
2. Based on your gender, body weight, and run time, use the regression equation designed for college students (18–29 yr) to determine your estimated VO_{2max}.
3. Record your test results and normative rating on Chart 7–1.

1.5 mile run regression equation*:

$$VO_{2max}\ (ml·kg^{-1}·min^{-1}) = 88.02 + (3.716 \times G)$$
$$- (0.1656 \times BW) - (2.767 \times T)$$

Where:
G = Gender (0 = female; 1 = male)
BW = Body weight (kg)
T = Elapsed run time (min)

Computation example: What is the estimated VO_{2max} ($ml·kg^{-1}·min^{-1}$) of a college male who is 19 years old, has a body weight of 175 lbs, and ran the 1.5 mile run in 8:07 min:sec? Show your work.

1. Convert this person's body weight from pounds to kilograms:

$$175\,lbs \times \frac{1\,kg}{2.2\,lbs} = 79.54\,kg$$

*Source: George et al. (March 1993).

ASSESSMENT OF OVERALL PHYSICAL FITNESS

139

2. Convert his jog time from a 00:00 value to a 00.00 value.

$$7 \, \text{seconds} \times \frac{1 \, \text{minute}}{60 \, \text{seconds}} = 0.116 \, \text{minutes}$$

3. Compute this person's estimated VO_{2max} with the following regression equation:

$$VO_{2max} \, (\text{ml} \cdot \text{kg}^{-1} \cdot \text{min}^{-1}) = 88.02 + (3.716 \times G) \\ - (0.1656 \times BW) - (2.767 \times T)$$

$$VO_{2max} \, (\text{ml} \cdot \text{kg}^{-1} \cdot \text{min}^{-1}) = 88.02 + (3.716 \times 1) \\ - (0.1656 \times 79.54) - (2.767 \times 8.116)$$

$$VO_{2max} \, (\text{ml} \cdot \text{kg}^{-1} \cdot \text{min}^{-1}) = 88.02 + (3.716) \\ - (13.17) - (22.45)$$

$$VO_{2max} = 56.11 \, \text{ml} \cdot \text{kg}^{-1} \cdot \text{min}^{-1}$$

Fitness Level: Excellent (See Table 5–1).

YMCA Submaximal Cycle Ergometer Protocol

1. Record your name, age, and weight on Chart 7–2. Also calculate and record your predicted maximum heart rate (220–age).
2. Use a calibrated cycle ergometer. Adjust the seat height so the knee is slightly bent when the pedal is in the down position. Record the seat height on Chart 7–2.
3. Have a partner administer the YMCA test protocol as outlined in Figure 7–1. The initial work rate should be set at 150 kgm·min⁻¹ (25 watts). Pedal speed should equal 50 rpm. Heart rates should be measured within the last minute of each stage. Adjust the work load according to each end-stage HR (see Figure 7–1). Note that the intent is to perform only one additional exercise stage beyond the point where a HR of at least 110 bpm is achieved. Thus, if a HR of 123 bpm were realized in the first stage, only one additional 3-minute stage should be performed; likewise a HR of 118 bpm in the third stage would necessitate only one more 3-minute stage.

    The YMCA test is designed to require about 6–12 minutes of time (i.e., a minimum of two stages to a maximum of four stages).
4. Record your tests results in Chart 7–2. Plot the data (work rate versus heart rate) from 2–3 exercise stages. Use a straightedge to establish a line of best fit between your data points and extrapolate to intersect the predicted maximum heart rate line (see Figure 7–2). Directly below this point of intersection, along the bottom of Chart 7–2, will be your corresponding VO_{2max} estimation score. See example in Figure 7–2.
5. Record your test results and normative rating on Chart 7–1.

Computation example: What would be the estimated VO_{2max} (ml·kg⁻¹·min⁻¹) of a 40-yr-old male who weighs 80 kg and performed 3 stages of the YMCA protocol? Assume a HR (bpm) and work rate (kgm·50 (third stage). In addition, assume a predicted maximum heart rate of 180 bpm.

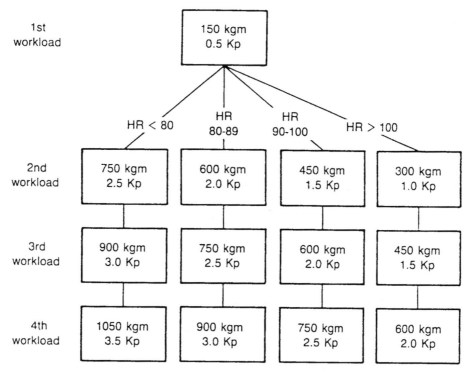

1st workload	150 kgm 0.5 Kp			
	HR < 80	HR 80-89	HR 90-100	HR > 100
2nd workload	750 kgm 2.5 Kp	600 kgm 2.0 Kp	450 kgm 1.5 Kp	300 kgm 1.0 Kp
3rd workload	900 kgm 3.0 Kp	750 kgm 2.5 Kp	600 kgm 2.0 Kp	450 kgm 1.5 Kp
4th workload	1050 kgm 3.5 Kp	900 kgm 3.0 Kp	750 kgm 2.5 Kp	600 kgm 2.0 Kp

Directions:

1. Set the first workload at 150 kgm/min (0.5 Kp).
2. If the HR in the third min is

   - less than (<) 80, set the second load at 750 kgm (2.5 Kp);
   - 80 to 89, set the second load at 600 kgm (2.0 Kp);
   - 90 to 100, set the second load at 450 kgm (1.5 Kp);
   - greater than (>) 100, set the second load at 300 kgm (1.0 Kp).

3. Set the third and fourth (if required) loads according to the loads in the columns below the second loads.

Figure 7–1. Guidelines for YMCA Cycle Ergometer Protocol. Source: *The Y's Way to Physical Fitness* (3rd edition; 1989). YMCA of the USA, 101 N. Wacker Drive, Chicago, IL 60606.

1. Refer to the example in Figure 7–2. Notice that the three points were plotted according to the heart rate versus work rate data. Also note that an extrapolation line (dashed line) was drawn up to the maximum heart rate line.

2. Directly below this point of intersection, along the bottom of the graph, is the VO_{2max} estimation score, which equals 1.6 $1 \cdot min^{-1}$. Observe that an estimated maximum work rate of 650 $kgm \cdot min^{-1}$ is also recorded. Can you see how this value was determined?

3. Convert the estimated VO_{2max} score of 1.6 $1 \cdot min^{-1}$ to $ml \cdot kg \cdot 1 \cdot min^{-1}$:

$$VO_{2max} = 1.6 \text{ L/min} \times 1000 \text{ ml/L} = 1600 \text{ ml} \cdot min^{-1}$$

$$1600 \text{ ml/min} \div 80 \text{ kg} = 20 \text{ ml} \cdot kg^{-1} \cdot min^{-1}$$

Fitness Level: Fair (See Table 5–1).

Hand-grip test

1. Instructions for this test are found in Chapter 2.
2. Record your test results and normative rating on Chart 7–1.

NAME Example Male   AGE 40   WEIGHT 176 LB 80 KG   SEAT HEIGHT 8

PREDICTED MAX HR _____

	DATE	1st WORKLOAD HR USED	2nd WORKLOAD HR USED	3rd WORKLOAD HR USED	MAX WORKLOAD	MAX O₂(L/min)	MAX O₂(mL/kg)
TEST 1	1-4-88	150/105	300/120	450/145	650	1.6	$\frac{1600}{80} = 20$
TEST 2							
TEST 3							

DIRECTIONS

1. Plot the HR of the 2 workloads versus the work (kgm/min).

2. Determine the subject's max HR line by subtracting subject's age from 220 and draw a line across the graph at this value.

3. Draw a line through both points and extend to the max HR line for age.

4. Drop a line from this point to the baseline and read the predicted max workload and O₂ uptake.

WORKLOAD (kgm/min)	150	300	450	600	750	900	1050	1200	1350	1500	1650	1800	1950	2100
MAX O₂ UPTAKE (L/m)	0.6	0.9	1.2	1.5	1.8	2.1	2.4	2.8	3.2	3.5	3.8	4.2	4.6	5.0
KCAL USED (kcal/m)	3.0	4.5	6.0	7.5	9.0	10.5	12.0	14.0	16.0	17.5	19.0	21.0	23.0	25.0
APPROX MET LEVEL (for 132 lb)	3.3	4.7	6.0	7.3	8.7	10.0	11.3	12.7	14.0	15.3	16.7	18.0	19.3	20.7
APPROX MET LEVEL (for 176 lb)	3.0	4.0	5.0	6.0	7.0	8.0	9.0	10.0	11.0	12.0	13.0	14.0	15.0	16.0

Figure 7–2. Sample Graph for the YMCA Cycle Ergometer Test. Source: *The Y's Way to Physical Fitness* (3rd edition; 1989). YMCA of the USA, 101 N. Wacker Drive, Chicago, IL 60606.

I RM Bench Press and Leg Press

1. Estimate your 1 RM weight for the bench press.
2. Select a warm-up weight that is about 50 percent of your estimated 1 RM. Bench press this weight several times as a warm up. Progressively increase the weight (i.e., 5–10 lb increments) until you can only lift the weight once with maximal effort. Be sure to rest at least one minute between repetitions.
3. Record your 1 RM on Chart 7–1.
4. Based on your 1 RM data, determine your strengh-to-weight ratio and normative rating (Table 7–1). Show your work and attach.
5. Repeat steps 1–4 for the leg press.
6. Record your results and normative rating on Chart 7–1.

Traditional and Modified Sit-and-Reach Tests

1. Remove your shoes and stretch/warm up as desired.
2. Perform one of the sit-and-reach flexibility tests as outlined in Chapter 3.
3. Record your results and normative rating on Chart 7–1.

Table 7–1
Relative Strength Norm Chart
Strength-to-Weight Ratios

	1 RM Bench Press		1 RM Leg Press	
Category	Male	Female	Male	Female
Excellent	>1.25	>0.77	>2.07	>1.62
Good	1.17–1.25	0.72–0.77	2.00–2.07	1.54–1.62
Average	0.97–1.16	0.59–0.71	1.83–1.99	1.35–1.53
Fair	0.88–0.96	0.53–0.58	1.65–1.82	1.26–1.34
Poor	<0.88	<0.53	<1.65	<1.26

Source: Institute for Aerobic Research, Dallas Texas (Ages 20–29).

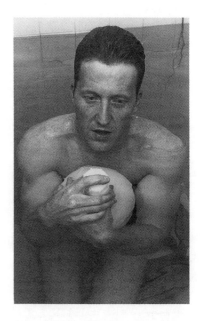

Σ3 Skinfold Test

1. With your partner, measure the three skinfold sites necessary to predict body density and percent body fat (see Chapter 6).
2. Calculate your body density and percent body fat. Show work and attach.
3. Record your test results and normative rating on Chart 7–1.

Natant Hydrostatic Weighing

1. Get with a partner and find a place in the pool where the water level is about chest or shoulder height.
2. Hold the Natant system against your chest and breathe in and out 3–4 times.
3. Descend slowly in the water and assume a fetal position while underwater.
4. Exhale maximally! While underwater, continue to force out as much air as possible—don't hold any air back. *Note:* In order to expire completely, contract and relax your abdominal muscles several times during the final portion of your exhalation.
5. You must remain underwater at least 3–5 seconds after you have exhaled as much air as possible. This will allow your partner enough time to determine whether you're sinking or floating.
6. Continue the Natant procedure until you assume a neutral buoyant position—neither sinking nor floating (i.e., head approximately 4 inches below the surface; feet not touching bottom).
7. Your instructor will show you how to quantify your Natant measurement.
8. When you have completed the Natant procedure, record all test information in Chart 7–1. Be sure to record the water temperature (°C) in the appropriate space.

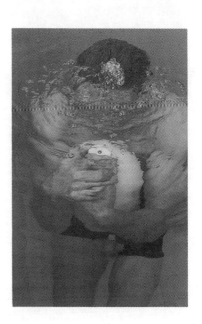

9. Use the Natant computer program and compute your body density and percent fat.
10. Record your test results and normative rating on Chart 7–1.

Note: To maximize the accuracy of your hydrostatic weighing test, you should avoid strenuous exercise the day of the test, standardize the amount of food eaten 24 hours before testing, maintain a normal hydration level (i.e., not be retaining water), and void immediately before your test. Be very strict in the administration of this test and make sure, through repeated trials, that neutral buoyancy is achieved and that full expirations are performed for each trial. Error on hydrostatic methods often comes from the subject not expiring his or her air properly.

Physical Best Physical Fitness Evaluation

The Physical Best program developed by AAHPERD provides a physical fitness test battery for youths aged 5 to 18 years. Outlined below are instructions for each test item as provided in the Physical Best manual. It is suggested that the test sequence be performed in the order presented below. If your instructor assigns you to perform these tests, use the health-related criterion standards for 18-year-olds in Tables 7–2 and 7–3. However, be aware that your actual standards may be somewhat different, assuming your age is significantly greater than 18 years.

Body Mass Index

1. Instructions for this measure are found in Chapter 6. Compute your BMI and record on Chart 7–3.
2. Refer to the appropriate Physical Best health-related standards (Table 7–2 or 7–3) to determine whether you passed this test item. Record your results on Chart 7–3.

Sum of Skinfolds Test

1. With your partner, measure the two skinfold sites necessary to estimate your body composition. Measure the triceps (see Chapter 6) and calf skinfold. To measure the calf skinfold, have your partner rest his or her right foot on a chair or stool (right knee should be flexed at about a 90° angle). The calf site is along the medial side (above the medial malleolus) at the maximum calf circumference. (A vertical skinfold should be taken.) Record your skinfold measures on Chart 7–3.
2. Sum the triceps and calf measures and refer to Table 7–2 or 7–3 to determine whether or not you satisfied the AAHPERD health-related standard. Note that no estimate of percent body fat is provided for this test item. Record your results on Chart 7–3.

Sit-Up Test

1. Lie on your back with knees flexed, feet on floor, and heels between 12 and 18 inches from the buttocks. The arms should be crossed on the chest with the hands on the opposite shoulder. Have your partner hold

Table 7–2
AAHPERD Health-Related Standards
Girls

Age	1-Mile Run (min)	Sum of Skinfolds (mm)	Body Mass Index	Sit and Reach* (cm)	Sit-Up (reps)	Pull-Up (reps)
5	14:00	16–36	14–20	25	20	1
6	13:00	16–36	14–20	25	20	1
7	12:00	16–36	14–20	25	24	1
8	11:00	16–36	14–20	25	26	1
9	11:00	16–36	14–20	25	28	1
10	11:00	16–36	14–21	25	30	1
11	11:00	16–36	14–21	25	33	1
12	11:00	16–36	15–22	25	33	1
13	10:30	16–36	15–23	25	33	1
14	10:30	16–36	17–24	25	35	1
15	10:30	16–36	17–24	25	35	1
16	10:30	16–36	17–24	25	35	1
17	10:30	16–36	17–25	25	35	1
18	10:30	16–36	18–26	25	35	1

*Note: Footline set at 23 cm; thus participants must stretch 2 cm beyond the footline to satisfy criterion.
Source: AAHPERD (1988).

Table 7–3
AAHPERD Health-Related Standards
Boys

Age	1-mile Run (min)	Sum of Skinfolds (mm)	Body Mass Index	Sit and Reach* (cm)	Sit-Up (reps)	Pull-Up (reps)
5	13:00	12–25	13–20	25	20	1
6	12:00	12–25	13–20	25	20	1
7	11:00	12–25	13–20	25	24	1
8	10:00	12–25	14–20	25	26	1
9	10:00	12–25	14–20	25	30	1
10	9:30	12–25	14–20	25	34	1
11	9:00	12–25	15–21	25	36	2
12	9:00	12–25	15–22	25	38	2
13	8:00	12–25	16–23	25	40	3
14	7:45	12–25	16–24	25	40	4
15	7:30	12–25	17–24	25	42	5
16	7:30	12–25	18–24	25	44	5
17	7:30	12–25	18–25	25	44	5
18	7:30	12–25	18–26	25	44	5

*Note: Footline set at 23 cm; thus, participants must stretch 2 cm beyond the footline to satisfy criterion.
Source: AAHPERD (1988).

Table 7–4
Women's AFROTC Body Weight Standards

Ht (inches)	Minimum Wt (lbs)	Maximum Wt (lbs)	Ht (inches)	Minimum Wt (lbs)	Maximum Wt (lbs)
60.0	92	136.0	70.5	119	175.00
60.5	92	137.0	71.0	122	177.0
61.0	95	138.0	71.5	122	179.5
61.5	95	139.5	72.0	125	182.0
62.0	97	141.0	72.5	125	185.0
62.5	97	141.5	73.0	128	188.0
63.0	100	142.0	73.5	128	191.0
63.5	100	144.0	74.0	130	194.0
64.0	103	146.0	74.5	130	196.5
64.5	103	148.0	75.0	133	199.0
65.0	106	150.0	75.5	133	202.0
65.5	106	152.5	76.0	136	205.0
66.0	108	155.0	76.5	136	207.5
66.5	108	158.0	77.0	139	210.0
67.0	111	159.0	77.5	139	212.5
67.5	111	161.5	78.0	141	215.0
68.0	114	164.0	78.5	141	218.0
68.5	114	166.0	79.0	144	221.0
69.0	117	168.0	79.5	144	223.5
69.5	117	170.5	80.0	147	226.0
70.0	119	173.0	80.5	147	229.0

Note: For every inch under 60 inches, subtract 2 pounds from the maximum allowable weight; for every inch over 80 inches, add 6 pounds to the maximum allowable weight. Official weigh-ins may be delayed 10 days for women who are experiencing their menstrual cycle.

Source: Air Force ROTC (1992).

your feet. The up position is completed when your elbows touch your thighs; the down position is completed when your mid-back makes contact with the floor.

2. Perform as many sit-ups as possible in one minute. Have your partner count the number of complete repetitions. Rest between sit-ups is allowed in either the up or down position.
3. Record the number of sit-ups completed on Chart 7–3.
4. Refer to the appropriate Physical Best health-related standards (Table 7–2 or 7–3) to determine whether you passed this test item. Record your results on Chart 7–3.

Pull-Up Test

1. Hang from a bar using an overhand (palms forward) grip. Keep your arms and legs fully extended, with your feet above the floor.
2. From a hanging position, raise your body with the arms until the chin is above the bar; then lower the body again to the fully extended position.

Table 7–5
Men's AFROTC Body Weight Standards

Ht (inches)	Minimum Wt (lbs)	Maximum Wt (lbs)	Ht (inches)	Minimum Wt (lbs)	Maximum Wt (lbs)
60.0	100	153.0	70.5	123	196.5
60.5	100	154.0	71.0	127	199.0
61.0	102	155.0	71.5	127	202.5
61.5	102	156.5	72.0	131	205.0
62.0	103	158.0	72.5	131	208.0
62.5	103	159.0	73.0	135	211.0
63.0	104	160.0	73.5	135	214.5
63.5	104	162.0	74.0	139	218.0
64.0	105	164.0	74.5	139	221.0
64.5	105	166.5	75.0	143	224.0
65.0	106	169.0	75.5	143	227.0
65.5	106	171.5	76.0	147	230.0
66.0	107	174.0	76.5	147	233.0
66.5	107	176.5	77.0	151	236.0
67.0	111	179.0	77.5	151	239.0
67.5	111	181.5	78.0	153	242.0
68.0	115	184.0	78.5	153	245.0
68.5	115	186.5	79.0	157	248.0
69.0	119	189.0	79.5	157	251.0
69.5	119	191.5	80.0	161	254.0
70.0	123	194.0	80.5	161	257.0

Note: For every inch under 60 inches, subtract 2 pounds from the maximum allowable weight; for every inch over 80 inches, add 6 pounds to the maximum allowable weight.
Source: Air Force ROTC (1992).

Table 7–6
AFROTC Performance-Related Standards
1.5-Mile Run

Age (yr)	Male (min:sec)	Female (min:sec)
17–29	12:00	14:24
30 or older	12:30	14:52

Mandatory time adjustments for altitude: At 5,000 ft add 30 seconds; at 8,000 ft add 1 minute; at 12,000 ft add 2 minutes to standards.
Source: Air Force ROTC (1992).

3. Repeat as many times as possible. There is no time limit.
4. Record the number of pull-ups completed on Chart 7–3.
5. Refer to the appropriate Physical Best health-related standards (Table 7–2 or 7–3) to determine whether you passed this test item. Record your results on Chart 7–3.

Sit-and-Reach Test

1. Warm up the low back and hamstrings prior to testing with slow, sustained, steady (no bobbing) stretching.
2. Perform the traditional sit-and-reach test as explained in Chapter 3. You are allowed four trials. Each trial should be held at least one second.
3. Record your best sit-and-reach score on Chart 7–3.
4. Refer to the appropriate Physical Best health-related standards (Table 7–2 or 7–3) to determine whether you passed this test item. Note that the footline for the Physical Best program is set at 23 cm; thus if your sit-and-reach box has a different footline position, you will need to adjust the health-related stndard accordingly (i.e., if footline = 25 cm, adjusted standard would equal 27 cm and not 25 cm). Record your results on Chart 7–3.

1-Mile Run Test

1. Warm up prior to the test.
2. Run 1.0 mile as fast as possible over a level surface (i.e., track). Have your partner record your time. Pace yourself so you can sustain the fastest pace over the full distance covered.
3. Record your time on Chart 7–3.
4. Refer to the appropriate Physical Best health-related standards (Table 7–2 or 7–3) to determine whether you passed this test item. Record your results on Chart 7–3.

AFROTC Physical Fitness Test Battery

The United States Air Force ROTC (AFROTC) has developed a battery of physical fitness tests designed to evaluate the physical competence of applicants and enlisted personnel. Specific performance-related criterion-reference standards (Tables 7–6 and 7–7) reflect the minimum level of physical fitness required for military operations.

Outlined below are instructions for each test item as provided in AFROTC operations manual. The pull-ups or flexed arm hang, long jump, push-ups, sit-ups, and 600-yard run should be performed in this order and all should be completed in a 15-minute period. The 1.5-mile run can be performed on a separate day. Warm-up exercises are encouraged before performance of the 15-minute test protocol or 1.5-mile run.

Body Weight

1. Have your partner weigh you to the nearest quarter pound. Record on Chart 7–4.
2. Have your partner measure your height to the nearest quarter inch. Record on Chart 7–4.
3. Based on the appropriate body weight standards (Table 7–4 or 7–5) ascertain whether or not you are between the minimal and maximal allowable body weight. Record on Chart 7–4.

1.5-Mile Run Test

1. Run 1.5 miles as fast as possible over a level surface (i.e., track). Have your partner record your time.
2. Based on your age and gender, determine whether or not you satisfy the performance standard (Table 7–6).
3. Record your results on Chart 7–4.

Pull-Up Test

Men

1. Palms may face in or out with hands approximately a shoulder width apart. Chin must clear bar at a 90-degree angle with the neck.
2. From a hanging position, raise your body with the arms until the chin is above the bar; then lower the body again to the fully extended position. Kicking or swaying the body is not allowed.
3. The exercise is completed when maximum score is achieved (19 repetitions) or when there is a failure to complete an attempted pull-up or when resting for an extended period of time (i.e., in excess of 5 seconds).
4. Record the number of pull-ups completed on Chart 7–4.
5. Based on the men's score sheet (Table 7–7), determine the number of points earned for this test. Also determine whether you meet the minimum requirement for this test. Record on Chart 7–4.

Flexed Arm Hang

Women

1. Climb a step ladder until your chin is above the pull-up bar. Assume an overhand (palms forward) grip with the hands about shoulder width.
2. Have your partner move the step ladder away from under your feet and time your test. You should hold the flexed arm hang position as long as possible. Be sure the chin never rests on the bar or that the head tilts backward to keep the chin above the bar.
3. The test is completed when a maximum score is achieved (42 seconds), when the chin rests on the bar, or when the chin falls below the bar or the head tilts backward to keep the chin above the bar.
4. Record the time of your test in seconds on Chart 7–4.
5. Based on the women's score sheet (Table 7–8), determine the number of points earned for this test. Also determine whether you meet the minimum requirement for this test. Record your results on Chart 7–4.

Standing Long Jump

1. Toes should be positioned close to but not touching the starting line. Both feet should leave the ground simultaneously.
2. Jump as far as possible.
3. First jump may be counted as practice. Two jumps are allowed. If first jump is satisfactory, second jump can be optional.
4. Measure the distance jumped (in inches) from start line to point of contact. Record your score on Chart 7–4.
5. Based on the appropriate score sheet (Table 7–7 or 7–8), determine the number of points earned for this test. Also determine whether you meet the minimum requirement for this test. Record on Chart 7–4.

Push-Up Test

1. Feet and hands should be no more than shoulder width. Avoid excessive arching of the body (positive or negative arch). Body position is the same for both males and females.
2. Lower your body until your sternum touches your partner's knuckles (partner's fist on the ground with the four finger knuckles upward). Lift your body until the arms are completely extended. At no time should any part of the body be allowed to rest on the ground, other than hands and toes. Count only complete push-ups.
3. The test is completed when the maximum score is achieved (70 for males, 37 for females), when rest in the up position exceeds 5 seconds, or at failure to complete attempted push-up.
4. Based on the appropriate score sheet (Table 7–7 or 7–8), determine the number of points earned for this test. Also determine whether you meet the minimum requirement for this test. Record on Chart 7–4.

Sit-Up Test

1. Lie on your back with knees flexed, feet on floor, and heels no further than shoulder width apart. Lock your hands behind your head throughout exercise. Body position is the same for both males and females.
2. Perform as many sit-ups as possible in two minutes. In up position, touch either elbow to knee; in down position, shoulder blades must touch surface. No resting is allowed in the down position.
3. The test is completed after the two-minute time limit or when the maximum score is reached (88 for males, 79 for females), or when rest in up position exceeds 5 seconds, or at failure to complete attempted sit-up.
4. Record the score on Chart 7–4.
5. Based on the appropriate score sheet (Table 7–7 or 7–8), determine the number of points earned for this test. Also determine whether you meet the minimum requirement for this test. Record on Chart 7–4.

600-Yard Run Test

1. Run 600 yards as fast as possible over level terrain.
2. Have your partner time your run.
3. Record your results on Chart 7–4.
4. Based on the appropriate score sheet (Table 7–7 or 7–8), determine the number of points earned for this test. Also determine whether you meet the minimum requirement for this test. Record on Chart 7–4.

Computation of Results

1. Add up the points earned for the pull-ups or flexed arm hang, standing long jump, push-ups, sit-ups, and 600-yard run. Record on Chart 7–4. A score of at least 180 points is required, along with a minimum passing score in any four of the five events.
2. Participants should also satisfy the body weight and 1.5-mile run requirements to pass the test.
3. Indicate on Chart 7–4 whether or not you passed the test.

Table 7–7
Men's AFROTC Score Sheet

Pull-Ups		Long Jump		Push-Ups		Sit-Ups		600-Yd Run	
Reps	Pts	Inches	Pts	Reps	Pts	Reps	Pts	Seconds	Pts
19	100	104	100	70	100	88	100	95	100
18	99	103	97	69	96	87	94	96	97
17	94	102	93	68	93	86	92	97	94
16	89	101	90	67	92	85	91	98	91
15	83	100	86	66	91	84	89	99	88
14	78	99	83	65	88	83	87	100	85
13	73	98	80	64	86	82	86	101	82
12	67	97	76	63	84	81	84	102	79
11	62	96	73	62	83	80	83	103	76
10	57	95	69	61	81	79	81	104	73
9	51	94	66	60	79	78	79	105	70
8	46	93	63	59	77	77	78	106	67
7	·41	92	59	58	75	76	76	107	64
6	36	91	56	57	74	75	75	108	61
5	30	90	52	56	72	74	73	109	58
** 4	25	89	49	55	70	73	71	110	55
3	20	88	45	54	68	72	70	111	52
2	14	87	41	53	66	71	68	112	49
1	9	86	37	52	65	70	67	113	46
		85	33	51	63	69	65	114	43
		84	29	50	61	68	63	115	40
		**83	25	49	59	67	62	116	37
		82	21	48	57	66	60	117	34
		81	19	47	56	65	59	118	31
		80	17	46	54	64	57	119	29
		79	15	45	52	63	55	120	27
		78	13	44	50	62	54	**121	25
		77	11	43	48	61	52	122	22
		76	9	42	47	60	51	123	19
		75	7	41	45	59	49	124	16
		74	5	40	43	58	47	125	13
		73	2	39	41	57	46	126	10
				38	39	56	44	127	8
				37	38	55	43	128	6
				36	36	54	41	129	4
				35	34	53	39	130	2
				34	32	52	38		
				33	30	51	36		
				32	29	50	35		
				31	27	49	33		
				**30	25	48	31		
				29	23	47	30		
				28	21	46	28		
				27	18	45	27		
				26	16	**44	25		
				25	14	43	23		
				24	12	42	21		
				23	10	41	19		
				22	7	40	17		
				21	5	39	15		
				20	3	38	13		
						37	11		
						36	9		
						35	7		
						34	5		
						33	3		

** = Performance-related criterion standard
Source: Air Force ROTC (1992).

Table 7–8
Women's AFROTC Score Sheet

Flexed Arm Hang		Long Jump		Push-Ups		Sit-Ups		600-Yd Run	
Seconds	Pts	Inches	Pts	Reps	Pts	Reps	Pts	Seconds	Pts
42	100	84	100	37	100	79	100	113	100
41	97	83	96	36	97	78	98	114	97
40	94	82	92	35	94	77	96	115	94
39	91	81	88	34	91	76	94	116	91
38	88	80	85	33	88	75	92	117	88
37	85	79	82	32	85	74	90	118	85
36	82	78	79	31	82	73	88	119	82
35	79	77	76	30	79	72	86	120	79
34	76	76	73	29	76	71	84	121	77
33	73	75	70	28	73	70	82	122	75
32	71	74	67	27	70	69	80	123	73
31	69	73	64	26	67	68	78	124	71
30	67	72	61	25	64	67	76	125	69
29	65	71	58	24	61	66	74	126	67
28	63	70	55	23	58	65	72	127	65
27	61	69	52	22	55	64	70	128	63
26	59	68	49	21	52	63	68	129	61
25	57	67	46	20	49	62	66	130	59
24	55	66	43	19	46	61	64	131	57
23	53	65	40	18	43	60	62	132	55
22	51	64	37	17	41	59	60	133	53
21	49	63	34	16	39	58	58	134	51
20	47	62	31	15	37	57	56	135	49
19	45	61	28	14	35	56	54	136	47
18	43	**60	25	13	33	55	52	137	45
17	41	59	21	12	31	54	50	138	43
16	39	58	17	11	29	53	48	139	41
15	37	57	13	10	27	52	46	140	39
14	35	56	9	**9	25	51	44	141	37
13	33	55	5	8	23	50	42	142	35
12	31	54	2	7	20	49	40	143	33
11	29			6	18	48	38	144	31
10	27			5	15	47	36	145	29
**9	25			4	12	46	34	146	27
8	23			3	9	45	32	**147	25
7	20			2	6	44	30	148	23
6	18			1	3	43	28	149	21
5	15					42	26	150	19
4	12					**41	25	151	17
3	9					40	21	152	15
2	6					39	18	153	13
1	3					38	15	154	11
						37	12	155	9
						36	9	156	7
						35	6	157	5
						34	3	158	3
								159	1

** = Performance-related criterion standard
Source: Air Force ROTC (1992).

Name:_____ Date:_____

Assessment of Overall Physical Fitness
Assignment

Age:_____ yrs   Gender: Male ☐   Female ☐   Time of Day:_____ AM/PM

Weight: _____ lbs, _____ kg Height _____ feet/inches

Resting heart rate: _____ bpm

Resting blood pressure: _____ SBP (mmHg)/ _____ DBP (mmHg)

Chart 7–1
**Overall Physical Fitness Assessment
Data Sheet**

Check the tests assigned to perform:

☐ Astrand cycle test	☐ 1 RM bench press test
☐ Rockport walking test	☐ 1 RM leg press test
☐ George-Fisher jogging test	☐ Traditional sit & reach test
☐ Treadmill jogging test	☐ Modified sit & reach test
☐ Forest Service step test	☐ ∑3 Skinfold test
☐ 1.5-mile run	☐ Natant hydrostatic weighing test
☐ YMCA Cycle Test	☐ Other:_____
☐ Hand-grip test	

Astrand cycle test:

Ending work rate _____ kgm/min

Ending heart rate _____ bpm

VO_{2max} _____ ml·kg^{-1}·min^{-1} (age adjusted)

Normative rating: _____

Rockport walking test:

Elapsed walk time _____ min:sec

Elapsed walk time _____ min

Ending heart rate _____ bpm

VO_{2max} _____ ml·kg^{-1}·min^{-1}

Normative rating _____

Chart 7–1 (continued)
Overall Physical Fitness Assessment
Data Sheet

George-Fisher jogging test:

Elapsed jog time _____ min:sec

Elapsed jog time _____ min

Ending heart rate _____ bpm

VO_{2max} _____ $ml \cdot kg^{-1} \cdot min^{-1}$

Normative rating _____

Treadmill jogging test

Treadmill speed _____ mph (level grade)

Ending heart rate _____ bpm

VO_{2max} _____ $ml \cdot kg^{-1} \cdot min^{-1}$

Normative rating _____

Forest Service step test:

Ending heart rate _____ beats

VO_{2max} _____ $ml \cdot kg^{-1} \cdot min^{-1}$

Normative rating _____

1.5-mile run test:

Elapsed run time _____ min:sec

Elapsed run time _____ min

VO_{2max} _____ $ml \cdot kg^{-1} \cdot min^{-1}$

Normative rating _____

YMCA Cycle Test:

Ending work rate _____ kgm/min

Ending work rate _____ bpm

VO_{2max} _____ $L \cdot min^{-1}$

VO_{2max} _____ $ml \cdot kg^{-1} \cdot min^{-1}$

Normative rating _____

Hand-grip test:

Right hand _____ kg

Left hand _____ kg

Sum _____ kg

Normative rating _____

Chart 7–1 (continued)
Overall Physical Fitness Assessment
Data Sheet

1 RM bench press test:

Resistance _____ lbs _____ kg

Strength-to-weight ratio _____

Normative rating: _____

1 RM leg press test:

Resistance _____ lbs _____ kg

Strength-to-weight ratio _____

Normative rating: _____

Traditional sit & reach test:

Score _____ cm

Normative rating: _____

Modified sit & reach test:

Score _____ cm

Normative rating: _____

∑3 Skinfold test:

Triceps (females) _____ mm

Suprailium (females) _____ mm

Thigh (males and females) _____ mm

Chest (males) _____ mm

Abdomen (males) _____ mm

Sum _____ mm

Db _____ kg/L

%BF _____ %

Normative rating: _____

Natant Hydrostatic Weighing:

Water temperature _____ °C

Natant measurement _____

%BF _____ %

Normative rating: _____

Chart 7–2

YMCA Cycle Ergometer Test Maximum Physical Working Capacity Prediction

NAME _____

TEST 1
TEST 2
TEST 3

DATE _____

AGE _____ WEIGHT _____ LB _____ KG _____ SEAT HEIGHT _____

1st WORKLOAD HR USED _____
2nd WORKLOAD HR USED _____

MAX WORKLOAD _____

MAX O₂(L/min) _____

PREDICTED MAX HR _____

MAX O₂(mL/kg) _____

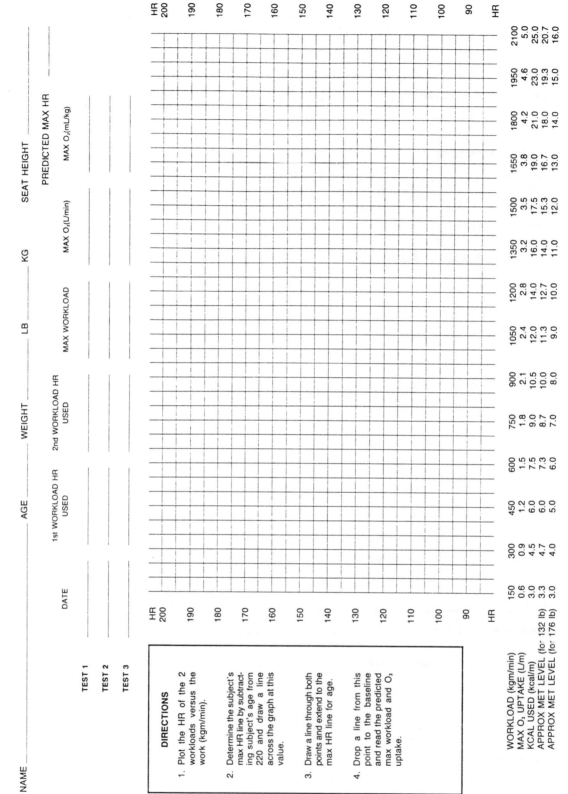

DIRECTIONS

1. Plot the HR of the 2 workloads versus the work (kgm/min).

2. Determine the subject's max HR line by subtracting subject's age from 220 and draw a line across the graph at this value.

3. Draw a line through both points and extend to the max HR line for age.

4. Drop a line from this point to the baseline and read the predicted max workload and O₂ uptake.

WORKLOAD (kgm/min)	150	300	450	600	750	900	1050	1200	1350	1500	1650	1800	1950	2100
MAX O₂ UPTAKE (L/m)	0.6	0.9	1.2	1.5	1.8	2.1	2.4	2.8	3.2	3.5	3.8	4.2	4.6	5.0
KCAL USED (kcal/m)	3.0	4.5	6.0	7.5	9.0	10.5	12.0	14.0	16.0	17.5	19.0	21.0	23.0	25.0
APPROX MET LEVEL (for 132 lb)	3.3	4.7	6.0	7.3	8.7	10.0	11.3	12.7	14.0	15.3	16.7	18.0	19.3	20.7
APPROX MET LEVEL (for 176 lb)	3.0	4.0	5.0	6.0	7.0	8.0	9.0	10.0	11.0	12.0	13.0	14.0	15.0	16.0

Source: *The Y's Way to Physical Fitness* (3rd edition: (1989). YMCA of the USA, 101 N. Wacker Drive, Chicago, IL 60606.

Chart 7–3
Physical Best Physical Fitness Test Battery

Data Sheet

Check the tests assigned to perform:
- ☐ Body mass index
- ☐ Sum of skinfolds
- ☐ Sit-up test
- ☐ Pull-up test
- ☐ Sit & reach test
- ☐ 1-mile run test

Body mass index:

Kg/m^2: _____

Health-related criterion satisfied: Yes / No

Sum of skinfolds:

Tricep: _____ mm

Calf: _____ mm

Sum: _____ mm

Health-related criterion satisfied: Yes / No

Sit-up test:

Score: _____ repetitions

Health-related criterion satisfied: Yes / No

Pull-up test:

Score: _____ repetitions

Health-related criterion satisfied: Yes / No

Sit & reach test:

Score: _____ cm

Health-related criterion satisfied: Yes / No

1-mile run test:

Elapsed run time: _____ min:sec

Health-related criterion satisfied: Yes / No

Chart 7–4
Air Force ROTC Physical Fitness Test Battery
Data Sheet

Check the tests assigned to perform:
- ☐ Body weight
- ☐ 1.5-mile run
- ☐ Pull-up test or flexed arm hang
- ☐ Standing long jump

- ☐ Push-up test
- ☐ Sit-up test
- ☐ 600-yard run

Body weight/height:
Current body weight: _____ lbs: height: _____ inches
Performance-related criterion satisfied: Yes / No

1.5-mile run test:
Elapsed run time: _____ min:sec
Performance-related criterion satisfied: Yes / No

Pull-up (males) / **Flexed arm hang** (females):
Score: _____ repetitions; _____ seconds
Point value: _____
Performance-related criterion satisfied: Yes / No

Standing long jump test:
Score: _____ inches
Point value: _____
Performance-related criterion satisfied: Yes / No

Push-up test:
Score: _____ repetitions
Point value: _____
Performance-related criterion satisfied: Yes / No

Sit-up test:
Score: _____repetitions
Point value: _____
Performance-related criterion satisfied: Yes / No

600-yard run test:
Elapsed run time: _____ seconds
Point value: _____
Performance-related criterion satisfied: Yes / No

Point total:
Pull-up test   _____
Standing long jump test   _____
Push-up test   _____
Sit-up test   _____
600-yard run   _____
Total score   _____

Criteria satisfied for overall test:
- ☐ Earned at least 180 points
- ☐ Achieved a minimum of any four of five event criterion standards
- ☐ Body weight criterion satisfied
- ☐ 1.5-mile run criterion satisfied

Passed test: Yes / No

Research Conclusions

1. Based on norm-reference standards, are you above average on the applicable physical fitness tests assigned by your instructor? Estimate what percent of your current level of fitness is attributed to your genetic endowment, exercise habits, and nutritional habits, respectively. Explain.

2. Based on AAHPERD health-related criterion-reference standards (18-year-old standards), do you satisfy the minimum score on the applicable physical fitness tests assigned by your instructor? Do you feel you possess a level of physical fitness that is associated with good health? Explain.

3. Based on AFROTC performance-related criterion-reference standards, do you satisfy the minimum score on the applicable physical fitness tests assigned by your instructor? Do you think the military should use health-related standards or performance-related standards to rate their applicants? Justify your answer.

4. With regard to overall physical fitness, what are your strengths and weaknesses? Are you content with your overall level of physical fitness?

5. Why would it be an advantage to improve and/or maintain your current level of physical fitness?

6. Outline several ways you could change your current lifestyle (exercise, nutritional habits, etc.) to improve your physical fitness. Be specific.

Name: _____   Date: _____

. . . .
Lab 7 Summary

Describe several ways the information learned in this lab can be applied to your chosen field of interest and/or your personal life. Be specific and provide practical examples.

8

Muscular Fatigue and Ischemia
. . . .
Pre-Laboratory Assignment

1. Define muscular fatigue.

2. Describe possible causes for muscular fatigue.

3. Define muscular ischemia.

4. Describe various ways to prevent muscular ischemia during exercise.

5. ❏ Check the box if you have read each research question and are familiar with the data collection procedures regarding each research question.

8

Muscular Fatigue and Ischemia

PURPOSE

The purpose of the this lab is to introduce concepts relating to muscular fatigue and muscular ischemia.

STUDENT LEARNING OBJECTIVES

1. Be able to define muscular fatigue and understand how to apply the knowledge learned from this lab to practical situations.
2. Be able to define muscular ischemia and describe how this condition can limit muscular strength and endurance.

NECESSARY EQUIPMENT

3 hand-grip dynamometers
2 sphygmomanometers (blood pressure cuffs)
Dumbbell weights

Muscular fatigue is the inability of the muscular system to maintain a given exercise intensity. The intensity and/or duration of exercise are the primary factors that induce the onset of muscular fatigue. Although the exact cause of muscular fatigue is not known, several possible causes include disruption of homeostasis within the neuromuscular pathway, including the upper and lower motor neurons; an inability to maintain adequate release of neurotransmitters at the neuromuscular junction; and compromising factors within the muscle itself. Muscular fatigue that results from a maximal exertion is probably related to insufficient ATP and creatine phosphate around the acto-myosin heads. Fatigue resulting from moderate to heavy exercise is likely due to the accumulation of waste products (CO_2, hydrogen ions) and the effects of such waste products on metabolic processes. Muscular fatigue that results from prolonged periods of light-to-moderate exercise is often caused by depletion of muscle glycogen and/or possible nervous system fatigue due to hypoglycemia (low blood sugar).

The athlete and the recreational enthusiast should understand how fatigue affects muscular fitness and what is required for a full recovery. Recovery infers that the body has reestablished its ability to maintain a desired exercise intensity. This means that the pre-exercise conditions within and surrounding the active tissue have been adequately restored. There are several factors that may affect the time of recovery, including the intensity and duration of the preceding exercise, the training status of the person, and/or the nutritional status of the person. During the recovery period, the fuel supply should be restored, the temperature of the body and active tissue brought back to normal, excessive waste products removed, and the cellular pH neutralized.

Muscular ischemia is defined as an inadequate supply of blood surrounding the muscle tissue. Muscular ischemia has a profound effect on muscular fitness since an insufficient amount of oxygen and nutrients reach the muscle and excessive waste products and metabolites are not transported away from the muscle cell. Certain types of exercises, equipment, and clothing may contribute to an ischemic state.

SELECTED REFERENCES

Barclay, J.K., and W. N. Stainsby (1975). The role of blood flow in limiting maximal metabolic rate in muscle. *Medicine and Science in Sports and Exercise*, 7:116–119.

Fitts, R. H., and J. O. Holloszy (1978). Effects of fatigue and recovery on contractile properties of frog muscle. *Journal of Applied Physiology* 45:899–902.

Fisher, A. G., and C. R. Jensen (1990). *Scientific Basis of Athletic Conditioning* (3rd edition). Philadelphia: Lea & Febiger, pp: 151–152.

Fox, E. L., R. W. Bowers, and M. L. Foss (1988). *The Physiological Basis of Physical Education and Athletics* (4th edition). Philadelphia: Saunders College Publishing, pp: 122–129.

Karsson, J. (1979). Localized muscular fatigue: Role of muscle metabolism and substrate depletion. *Exercise and Sport Sciences Review*, 7:1–42.

Lamb, D. R. (1984). *Physiology of Exercise: Responses and Adaptations* (2nd edition). New York: Macmillan Publishing Company, pp: 311–325.

McArdle, W. D., F. I. Katch, and V. L. Katch (1991). *Exercise Physiology: Energy, Nutrition, and Human Performance* (3rd edition). Philadelphia: Lea & Febiger, pp: 377.

Powers, S. K., and E. T. Howley (1990). *Exercise Physiology: Theory and Application to Fitness and Performance*. Dubuque, Iowa: Wm. C. Brown Publishers, pp: 418–421.

Wilmore, J. H., and D. L. Costill (1988). *Training for Sport and Activity: The Physiological Basis of the Conditioning Process* (3rd edition). Dubuque, Iowa: Wm. C. Brown Publishers, pp: 32–40, 196.

STATION 1
. . . .
Muscular Fatigue

Research Questions

1. Based on this experiment, how much recovery time was required before subjects attained 50% of their maximum strength? 100%? Summarize your results.

2. What impact does muscular fatigue have on maximum strength? Quantify your findings.

3. How does recovery time relate to intensity of effort in sports training?

Data Collection

1. Pre-treatment: Using a hand-grip dynamometer, determine the 1 RM for three members of your lab group. Record the results in Chart 8–1.
2. Treatment: Have subject #1 squeeze the hand-grip dynamometer at 100% effort for one minute. Have subject #2 squeeze the dynamometer at 50% effort (50% of 1 RM) for one minute. Have subject #3 rest. Have all three subjects start and stop this portion of the test at the same time.

   During the treatment, a member of the lab group should watch the dynamometer dial and assist subject #2 in maintaining the grip dynamometer tension at 50% of his or her 1 RM.

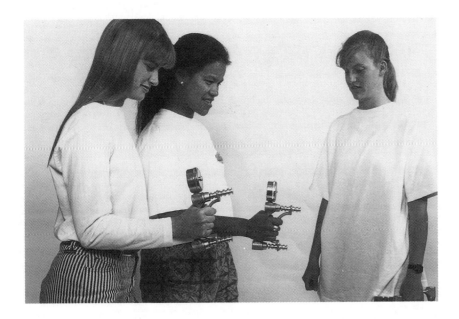

3. Post-treatment: Immediately following the conclusion of the one-minute treatment, reset the dynamometer dial and retest the maximum grip strength (1 RM) of all three subjects. Record the results in the 0:00 space in Chart 8–1.

4. In a post-treatment time period of 5 minutes, reassess the 1 RM grip strength of each subject every 30 seconds. Be sure to reset the dynamometer dial after each trial. Record the results of the post-treatment in Chart 8–2.

5. Plot your results on Chart 8–3 and be sure to:
   a. Plot *both* pre- and post-treatment data.
   b. Label the x and y axes.
   c. Provide an accurate scale for each axis.
   d. Connect the data points for each subject with a continuous line.
   e. Clearly label the data line of each subject.

Name: _____   Date: _____

Muscular Fatigue
Assignment

STATION 1

Chart 8–1 Data Sheet			
	Subject #1	Subject #2	Subject #3
Pre-treatment 1 RM (kg)	50.5	31.0	27.5
Treatment (1 minute)*	100%	50%	100%

*Subject #1 should squeeze grip dynamometer at 100% force for one minute; subject #2 should squeeze at 50% for one minute; subject #3 should rest for one minute.

Chart 8–2 Post-Treatment 1 RM Data Sheet			
Time (minutes)	Subject #1 1 RM (kg)	Subject #2 1 RM (kg)	Subject #3 1 RM (kg)
Immediate Post-Treatment	25.5	29.0	19.5
0:30	34.5	28.0	21.5
1:00	38.0	28.0	20.0
1:30	40.5	28.0	20.5
2:00	44.0	26.5	20.0
2:30	41.5	26.5	21.5
3:00	44.5	26.5	22.5
3:30	40.5	28.0	22.0
4:00	44.5	28.0	22.5
4:30	43.5	25.0	25.0
5:00	41.5	25.0	23.5

Chart 8–3
Plot of Strength vs Time

Research Conclusions

1. Based on this experiment, how much recovery time was required before subjects attained 50% of their maximum strength? 100%? Summarize your results.

The subjects were both able to obtain 50% of their maximum strength immediately after their one minute treatment. The 100% strength, however, was never obtained again even after five minutes.

2. What impact does muscular fatigue have on maximum strength? Quantify your findings.

Muscular fatigue causes the percentage of the maximum strength to drop drastically. In subject one, after muscular fatigue was obtained during the one minute treatment, the strength of the amount he could grip went from 50.5 kg to 25.5kg.

3. How does recovery time relate to intensity of effort in sports training?

The greater the intensity of a workout, the longer recovery time needed. This is due to the amount of PCr stores being depleated which causes a decrease in pH which in turn slows the production of ATP.

STATION 2
Muscular Ischemia

Research Questions

1. What impact does localized muscular ischemia have on relative muscular endurance? Describe your findings.

2. In athletics and recreational activities, when might localized ischemia occur? How could it be prevented and/or treated?

3. Describe two reasons why muscular ischemia should be prevented during training and athletic performance.

Data Collection

1. Use dumbbell weights to determine the maximum curl strength (1 RM) of the dominant arm for two members of your lab group. Record the results in Chart 8–4.
2. Secure a blood pressure cuff around the upper dominant arms of both subjects. Inflate one of the cuffs to a level of 150 mm Hg and leave the other empty.
3. Have the two subjects curl at a relative intensity of 70% of their maximum strength (i.e., 1 RM × 0.70 = exercise weight). Both subjects should perform their repetitions at the same cadence.
4. Have each subject continue this exercise until he or she can no longer maintain the set exercise cadence. Members of the lab group should count the total number of repetitions performed by each subject. Record results for each subject on Chart 8–4.

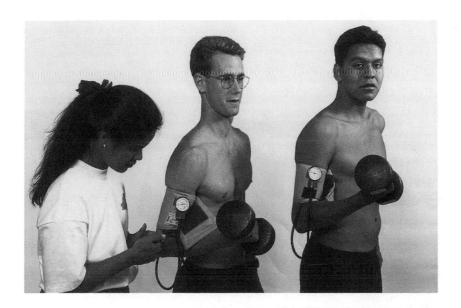

Name: _____ Date: _____

Muscular Ischemia
Assignment

STATION 2

Chart 8–4 Muscular Ischemia Data Sheet			
Treatment	1 RM (lbs)	70% of 1 RM (lbs)	Number of Repetitions
Subject with ischemia			
Subject without ischemia			

Research Conclusions

1. What impact does localized ischemia have on relative muscular endurance? Describe your findings.

2. In athletics and recreational activities, when might localized ischemia occur? How could it be prevented and/or treated?

3. Describe two reasons why muscular ischemia should be prevented during training and athletic performance.

. . . .
Lab 8 Summary

Describe several ways the information learned in this lab can be applied to your chosen field of interest and/or your personal life. Be specific and provide practical examples.

9

Muscular Power
· ·
Pre-Laboratory Assignment

1. Define muscular power.

2. List various factors that influence muscular power.

3. What is the Margaria–Kalamen Power Test score for a male who has a body weight of 95 kg, an elapsed time of 0.45 seconds, and a distance traveled of 1.03 meters?

4. What would be the cycle ergometer resistance, absolute and relative peak 5-second power output, absolute and relative mean 30-second power output, percentile rating, and fatigue index for a male subject who performed the Wingate Power Test. Assume he weighs 86 kg and pedal revolutions for each 5-second interval equaled 12, 10, 9, 7.5, 6, and 5.5 revolutions, respectively.

5. ☐ Check the box if you have read each research question and are familiar with the data collection procedures regarding each research question.

9
Muscular Power

PURPOSE
The purpose of this lab is to allow you to measure and evaluate muscular power.

STUDENT LEARNING OBJECTIVES
1. Be able to define muscular power.
2. Be able to describe how to measure this skill-related component of physical fitness using a simple field test.
3. Demonstrate the ability to compute and interpret the Wingate Power Test.

NECESSARY EQUIPMENT
Stairs (timing pads optional)
Cycle ergometer
Stop watch

Muscular power is defined as the amount of work performed per unit time or the rate at which force is exerted. A *powerful* movement usually infers that a maximal effort was put forth; however, the term *power* may also be used to describe submaximal movements. Maximal power is primarily determined by the total number and size of muscle fibers recruited; the motor unit fiber type (slow twitch versus fast twitch); body composition (% body fat); economy and skill of movement (training and technique); joint range of motion (flexibility); and coordination (applying force at the correct time). Because maximal power output involves explosive movements, the primary energy system to support this type of activity is anaerobic metabolism (stored ATP, CP-ATP, anaerobic glycolysis).

SELECTED REFERENCES
Adams, G. M. (1990). *Exercise Physiology Lab Manual.* Dubuque, Iowa: Wm. C. Brown Publishers, pp: 57–63, 85–112.

Bradley, A.L., and T.E. Ball (1992). The Wingate Test: effect of load on the power outputs of female athletes and nonathletes. *J. Appl. Sports Sci. Res.* 6(4):193–199.

Fisher, A. G., and C. R. Jensen (1990). *Scientific Basis of Athletic Conditioning* (3rd edition). Philadelphia: Lea & Febiger, pp: 254–257.

Fox, E. L., R. W. Bowers, and M. L. Foss (1988). *The Physiological Basis of Physical Education and Athletics* (4th edition). Philadelphia: Saunders College Publishing, pp: 64, 673–684.

Jacobs, I. (1980). The effects of thermal dehydration on performance of the Wingate Anaerobic Test. *International Journal of Sports Medicine* 1:21–24.

Lamb, D. R. (1984). *Physiology of Exercise: Responses and Adaptations* (2nd edition). New York: Macmillan Publishing Company, pp: 294–300.

Maud, P. J., and B. B. Shultz (1989). Norms for the Wingate Anaerobic Test with comparison to another similar test. *Research Quarterly for Exercise and Sport* 60(2):144–151.

Margaria, R., I. Aghemo, and E. Rovelli (1966). Measurement of muscular power (anaerobic) in man. *Journal of Applied Physiology* 21:1662–1664.

McArdle, W. D., F. I. Katch, and V. L. Katch (1991). *Exercise Physiology: Energy, Nutrition, and Human Performance* (3rd edition). Philadelphia: Lea & Febiger, pp: 201–204.

Powers, S. K., and E. T. Howley (1990). *Exercise Physiology: Theory and Application to Fitness and Performance.* Dubuque, Iowa: Wm. C. Brown Publishers, pp: 118–120.

Wilmore, J. H., and D. L. Costill (1988). *Training for Sport and Activity: The Physiological Basis of the Conditioning Process* (3rd edition). Dubuque, Iowa: Wm. C. Brown Publishers, pp: 369–373.

STATION 1
. . . .
Margaria-Kalamen Power Test

Research Questions

1. Do males and females have different levels of maximal power? If so, describe the difference and give several reasons why you would expect to see such findings.

2. Should norm charts for muscular power be gender specific? Defend your answer.

3. List at least two possible sources of measurement error that may have biased your findings. Would elimination of these errors change your answer to research question 1?

Data Collection

Each person in lab should perform the Margaria-Kalamen Power Test and/ or Wingate Power Test. When both tests are performed the same day, the Margaria-Kalamen Power Test should be performed before the Wingate Power Test.

Margaria-Kalamen Power Test
The Margaria-Kalamen Power Test requires the subject to run up a flight of stairs as fast as possible. The purpose of this test is to determine the anaerobic power output capabilities of primarily the legs and hips (plantar flexion, knee extension, and hip extension).

Instructions:

1. Locate a flight of stairs with at least 12 steps. Mark a starting point 6 meters in front of the first stair. Mark the third, sixth, and ninth stairs. If available, place timing mats on the third and ninth stairs so that stepping on the first mat (third stair) will start the clock, and stepping on the second mat (ninth stair) will turn off the clock. Record your elapsed time.
2. Jog toward the stairs from the starting position and climb the stairs as fast as possible. Climb three stairs per step, if possible.
    When automatic timing mats are not available, students can time each other with stop watches. Start and stop the watch when the runner steps on the third and ninth stairs, respectively.
3. Repeat the test at least three times or until you feel you have achieved your best time. Record your fastest time in hundredths of a second (00.00) on Chart 9–4.
4. Compute your power score. A computational example is provided below. Show your work in the space provided. Record your individual results on Chart 9–1. Refer to Table 9–1 to determine your power rating.

5. Record the results for each male and female on Chart 9–2. Compute the total and average male and female power score along with the corresponding power rating and also record on Chart 9–2.

Computation Example: What is the Margaria–Kalamen power test score for a female who has a body weight of 80 kg, an elapsed time of 0.55 seconds, and a distance traveled of 1.03 meters?

Power is computed using the following formula:

$$\text{Power (kgm/sec)} = \frac{f \times d}{t}$$

$$\text{Power} = \frac{80 \text{ kg} \times 1.03 \text{ m}}{0.55 \text{ sec}} = 149.8 \text{ kgm/sec}$$

Where: $f =$ Body weight in kilograms (kg)
  $d =$ Vertical distance between third and ninth stair in meters (m).
  $t =$ Time in hundredths of a second (s).
  (Use decimal, 0.00)

Note: Vertical distance (d) can be determined by measuring a single stair in meters and then multiplying by 6. This represents the entire vertical distance for all 6 stairs (between third and ninth stairs).

Power rating: Good. (See Table 9–1.)

Table 9–1
Margaria–Kalamen Power Test Norm Chart

Rating:	Men (kgm/sec)	Women (kgm/sec)
Poor	< 106	< 85
Fair	106–139	85–111
Average	140–175	112–140
Good	176–210	141–168
Excellent	> 210	> 168

Source: Fox (1988), for ages 20–30 years.

Name: _____   Date: _____

Margaria-Kalamen Power Test
Assignment

STATION 1

	Chart 9–1 **Muscular Power** **Individual Data Sheet**			
Force (kg)	Time (s)	Distance (m)	Power (kgm/sec)	Power Rating

Show your calculations:

Chart 9–2 **Muscular Power** **Class Data Sheet**			
Male		Female	
Subject	Power Score (kgm·min⁻¹)	Subject	Power Score (kgm·min⁻¹)
1		1	
2		2	
3		3	
4		4	
5		5	
6		6	
7		7	
8		8	
9		9	
10		10	
11		11	
12		12	
13		13	
14		14	
15		15	
Total		Total	
Average		Average	

Research Conclusions

1. Do males and females have different levels of maximal power? If so, describe the difference and give several reasons why you would expect to see such findings.

2. Should norm charts for muscular power be gender specific? Defend your answer.

3. List at least two possible sources of measurement error that may have biased your findings. Would elimination of these errors change your answer to question 1?

STATION 2
Wingate Power Test

Research Questions

1. Do your Wingate Power Test results equal those of a typical wrestler (males) or field hockey athlete (females)? See Table 9–2. Are you above the eightieth percentile in terms of your AMP and RMP scores on Chart 9–4? Discuss your findings.

2. Illustrate in graphical form your decline in relative peak power over the 30-second Wingate Power Test.

3. Describe at least two factors that may have caused a decline in power (fatigue) over the 30-second Wingate Test.

Data Collection

The Wingate Power Test involves pedaling a cycle ergometer at a maximal level of exertion (fastest pedal speed) for 30 seconds. This test is designed to measure the anaerobic power output for primarily knee extension (quadriceps muscle). Subject motivation is essential, and test results will not be valid unless subjects put forth maximal effort over the entire 30 second period. Accordingly, it is imperative that subjects perform at their maximal physical limits from the beginning to the end of the test.

Three measurements that indicate the anaerobic abilities of the muscle can be computed from the Wingate Power Test.

1. Peak 5-second power: This equals the highest 5-second power score during the 30-second test and should normally occur in the first 5 seconds of the test. A peak 5-second power score reflects the ability of the muscle to break down (utilize) ATP from primarily two sources: stored ATP and stored creatine phosphate (phosphagenic system).
2. Mean 30-second power: This equals the average power output of the muscle over the 30-second test. Because stored ATP and CP are depleted within the first 10 seconds, this measure primarily reflects ATP production via anaerobic glycolysis (degradation of glycogen).
3. Fatigue index: This reflects the ability of the muscle to resist fatigue. The fatigue index is equal to the difference between the highest 5-second power output and the lowest 5-second power output, divided by the highest 5-second power output (see formula below). A high score ($\geq 45\%$) indicates relatively low muscular endurance, whereas a low score ($\leq 30\%$) indicates the ability to resist muscular fatigue. It should be apparent that achieving an accurate fatigue index requires the subject to be motivated and pedal as fast as possible throughout the entire 30-second test.

In addition to the above three computations, relative scores for both peak 5-second power and mean 30-second power should also be calculated. To generate relative scores, simply divide the subject's power score (watts) by his or her body weight (kg). Relative scores are important because they provide an anaerobic power-to-weight ratio and can indicate the relative power of individuals with different body weights.

Instructions:

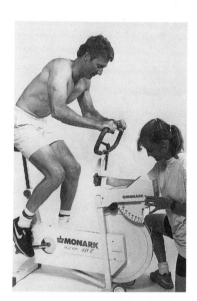

1. Organize the duties of your lab group. Assign lab members to (a) count pedal revolutions if an automatic counter is unavailable, (b) adjust the ergometer force, and (c) time the test.
2. Adjust the seat on the ergometer so that your subject's knees are nearly fully extended when the pedals are in the down position.
3. Have the subject warm up on a mechanically braked ergometer (Monark) for 2–4 minutes at an intensity to elicit a heart rate between 150–160 bpm. The cycling should be interspersed with 4–5 seconds of all out sprints to help the subject get a feel for the actual test.
4. After this warm up, the subject should rest for at least 2 minutes but not for more than 5 minutes.
5. On cue, the subject should pedal the ergometer as fast as possible. At the same time, the ergometer resistance should be increased to the predetermined resistance within 2–4 seconds. This resistance should equal 0.075 times body mass (kg). At the precise moment the optimal load has been reached, a count of the pedal revolutions should begin and continue for 30 seconds as the subject pedals as fast as possible.

   Pedal counts must be recorded every 5 seconds during this 30-second work phase, either electronically or by a reliable pair of observers. One observer should count the cumulative pedal revolutions out loud while the other records the results on Chart 9–3 every 5 seconds. Based on the cumulative pedal revolutions, the number of revolutions in each 5-second period can be determined.
6. Cool down: Have the subject continue pedaling at a light load for about 2–3 minutes following the test.
7. Calculate the peak anaerobic power, mean power output, and fatigue index. See the computation example below. Note that equations used to compute power are intended for Monark cycle ergometers or other comparable ergometers that have a flywheel equal to 6 meters per revolution.
8. Record your results on Chart 9–3.
9. Illustrate in graphical form the decline in relative peak power over the 30-second Wingate Power Test. Label the x axis as time (seconds) and the y axis as relative peak 5-second power (watts/kg). Draw a line to connect each plotted data point to illustrate trends in the data.

Computation example: What would be the cycle ergometer resistance, absolute and relative peak 5-second power output, absolute and relative mean 30-second power output, percentile rating, and fatigue index for a male who performed the Wingate Power Test? Assume he weighs 65 kg and pedal revolutions for each 5-second interval equaled 12, 10, 8.5, 7, 7, and 6.5 revolutions, respectively.

Cycle ergometer resistance:

$$65 \text{ kg} \times 0.075 = 4.87 \text{ kg or } 5.0 \text{ kg}$$

(*Note:* Round work loads to closest 0.5 kg)

Absolute peak 5-second power (APP):

$$\text{APP (watts)} = \text{load (kg)} \times \text{peak revolutions} \times 11.765$$

$$\text{APP} = 5 \text{ kg} \times 12 \text{ rev} \times 11.765 = 705.9 \text{ watts}$$

Relative peak 5-second power (RPP):

$$\text{RPP (watts/kg)} = \text{APP/kg body wt}$$

$$\text{RPP} = 705.9 \text{ watts/65 kg} = 10.86 \text{ watts/kg}$$

Absolute mean 30-second power (AMP):

$$\text{AMP (watts)} = \text{load (kg)} \times \text{average revolutions} \times 11.765$$

Average revolutions per 5-second interval =
$$12 + 10 + 8.5 + 7 + 7 + 6.5 = 51 \text{ revolutions}$$

$$51 \text{ rev/6 intervals of time} = 8.5 \text{ rev}$$

$$\text{AMP} = 5.0 \text{ kg} \times 8.5 \text{ rev} \times 11.765 = 500.0 \text{ watts}$$

Relative mean 30-second power (RMP):

$$\text{RMP (watts/kg)} = \text{AMP/kg}$$

$$\text{RMP} = 500.0 \text{ watts/65 kg} = 7.69 \text{ watts/kg}$$

Fatigue index (FI):

$$\text{FI (\%)} = \frac{\text{Highest peak 5-second power} - \text{lowest peak 5-second power}}{\text{Highest peak 5-second power}}$$

$$\text{FI} = \frac{705.9 \text{ watts} - 382.36 \text{ watts}}{705.9 \text{ watts}} = 0.4583 \text{ or } 45.83\%$$

$$\text{Lowest APP} = 5.0 \text{ kg} \times 6.5 \text{ rev} \times 11.765 = 382.36 \text{ watts}$$

Typical scores for APP, RPP, AMP, RMP, and FI for wrestling (males) and field hockey (females) are presented in Table 9-2. Percentile norms for AMP and RMP are illustrated on Table 9–3.

Table 9–2
Typical Power Scores for Wingate Power Test*

Group	APP (watts)	RPP (watts/kg)	AMP (watts)	RMP (watts/kg)	FI (%)
Wrestler (Male)	900	12.0	700	9.0	≤ 40%
Field Hockey (Female)	700	12.0	500	9.0	≤ 40%

APP = Absolute peak 5-second power (watts)
RPP = Relative peak 5-second power (watts/kg)
AMP = Absolute mean 30-second power (watts)
RMP = Relative mean 30-second power (watts/kg)

FI = Fatigue index (%)
*College students
Source: Bradley (1992) Jacobs (1980).

Table 9–3
Percentile Norms of AMP and RMP for Wingate Power Test*

Percentile Rank	Males		Females	
	AMP (watts)	RMP (watts/kg)	AMP (watts)	RMP (watts/kg)
95	676.6	8.63	483.0	7.52
90	661.8	8.24	469.9	7.31
85	630.5	8.09	437.0	7.08
80	617.9	8.01	419.4	6.95
75	604.3	7.96	413.5	6.93
70	600.0	7.91	409.7	6.77
65	591.7	7.70	402.2	6.65
60	576.8	7.59	391.4	6.59
55	574.5	7.46	386.0	6.51
50	564.6	7.44	381.1	6.39
45	552.8	7.26	376.9	6.20
40	547.6	7.14	366.9	6.15
35	534.6	7.08	360.5	6.13
30	529.7	7.00	353.2	6.03
25	520.6	6.79	346.8	5.94
20	496.1	6.59	336.5	5.71
15	484.6	6.39	320.3	5.56
10	470.9	5.98	306.1	5.25
5	453.2	5.56	286.5	5.07
Average	562.7	7.28	380.8	6.35
Standard Deviation	66.5	0.88	56.4	0.73
Minimum	441.3	4.63	235.4	4.53
Maximum	711.0	9.07	528.6	8.11

AMP = Absolute mean 30-second power (watts)
RMP = Relative mean 30-second power (watts/kg)

*Males (n = 60); Females (n = 69)
Source: Maud and Shultz (1989).

This table is reprinted with permission from the *Research Quarterly for Exercise and Sports*, vol. 60, no. 2 (June 1989). The *Research Quarterly for Exercise and Sport* is a publication of the American Alliance for Health, Physical Education, Recreation and Dance, 1900 Association Drive, Reston, VA 22091.

Name: _____ Date: _____

Lab 9 Summary

Describe several ways the information learned in this lab can be applied to your chosen field of interest and/or your personal life. Be specific and provide practical examples.

10
Measurement of Metabolic Rate
· ·
Pre-Laboratory Assignment

1. What would be the predicted BMR of a female who has a body weight of 156 lbs; a height of 5 feet, ten inches; and is 22 years old? Express your answer in kcal/day, kcal/min, $L O_2$/min, and $ml \cdot kg^{-1} \cdot min^{-1}$.

2. Describe several ways to minimize prediction errors when using the ACSM metabolic equations.

3. What is the estimated oxygen cost ($ml\ kg^{-1}\ min^{-1}$) and energy expenditure (kcal/min) of a treadmill jog of 5.5 mph and 10% grade? Assume a body mass of 73 kg.

4. What is the estimated oxygen cost (ml kg^{-1} min^{-1}) and energy expenditure (kcal/min) for leg cycle ergometry when a work rate of 750 kgm·min^{-1} is maintained? Assume a body weight of 86 kg.

5. ☐ Check the box if you have read each research question for this lab and are familiar with the data collection procedures regarding each research question.

10

Measurement of Metabolic Rate

PURPOSE

The purpose of this lab is to evaluate and compare observed versus estimated metabolic rate measurements.

STUDENT LEARNING OBJECTIVES

1. Be able to compute oxygen cost and energy expenditure values from prediction equations.
2. Be able to apply metabolic estimation equations to practical situations.

NECESSARY EQUIPMENT

Calculator
Metabolic cart
Mouthpiece(s) and noseclip
Treadmill
Cycle ergometer

The amount of energy the body uses each day is primarily dependent on two factors: basal metabolic rate and physical activity.

Basal Metabolic Rate

Basal metabolic rate (BMR) represents energy expended by the body (at rest) to maintain life and normal body functions (e.g., respiration, circulation, vital cellular needs). Surprisingly, BMR accounts for as much as 65–75% of daily kilo-calorie (kcal) expenditure. It is estimated that males and females expend an average of 1,500 and 1,200 kcals per day, respectively, just to maintain essential body function.

Numerous factors influence BMR. Among the most important are the size and composition of the body. For instance, larger individuals have more cells to service and support and consequently have a higher BMR than smaller individuals. In addition, muscle fibers require more energy to maintain (at rest) than do fat cells; hence, leaner individuals burn more calories over a 24-hr period than do fatter individuals of comparable size.

Measurement of BMR must be performed under stringent laboratory conditions. For example:

1. The person must not have eaten any food for at least 12 hours because digestion of food (thermogenesis) can significantly increase metabolic cost.
2. BMR must be measured when the person is completely rested but is still awake.
   a. Measurements should be made early in the morning following a night of restful sleep.
   b. No strenuous exercise should be performed for at least 24 hours before testing.
3. The person must be free of all psychic and physical disturbances (e.g., medications, drugs, depression, stress).

4. Room temperature must be comfortable and somewhere between 68° to 80° F.

Because the measurement of BMR requires careful control and subject preparation, resting metabolic rate (RMR) is frequently measured instead of BMR. The pre-test preparation for RMR measurements is to simply have the subject sit (or lie down) quietly for at least 10 minutes before testing. Accordingly, RMR will fluctuate more than BMR and will normally be a higher number. Typical resting metabolic rates are illustrated in Table 10–1.

There are several ways to measure BMR or RMR. The standard procedure employed by researchers is to use a whole-body calorimeter (metabolic chamber). A calorimeter is a large insulated chamber that can measure the amount of heat given off by the body. A metabolic chamber provides accurate, valid, and reliable test results; however, the equipment is expensive and difficult to use.

Fortunately, metabolic heat production is proportional to oxygen consumption. Accordingly, energy expenditure can be computed with an appropriate oxygen to kcalorie equivalent (i.e., 5 kcals/1 L O_2). A spirometer is often used to measure oxygen consumption at rest. Note that all observed measures of BMR or RMR should be corrected to STPD. (See Chapter 12 and Appendix C.)

Prediction of BMR

BMR can also be estimated with prediction equations. Outlined below are BMR prediction equations for both males and females. Predictor variables utilized to estimate BMR are body weight (kg), height (cm), and age.

Females:

$$\text{BMR (kcal/day)} = 655.1 + (9.56 \times \text{body weight;kg}) + (1.85 \times \text{height;cm}) - (4.68 \times \text{age;yr})$$

Table 10–1
Average Resting Metabolic Rates*

1.25 kcal·min⁻¹
0.25 L O_2·min⁻¹
3.5 ml·kg⁻¹·min⁻¹

*Values are corrected to STPD and represent typical RMR values over the entire population.

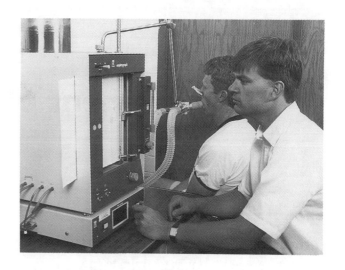

Males:

$$\text{BMR (kcal/day)} = 66.47 + (13.75 \times \text{body weight; kg}) + (5.0 \times \text{height; cm}) - (6.76 \times \text{age; yr})$$

Source: Harris and Benedict (1919).

Computation example: What would be the predicted BMR of a male who has a body weight of 200 lbs; a height of 6 feet, 5 inches; and is 27 years old? Express your answer in kcal/day, kcal/min, L O_2/min, and ml·kg⁻¹·min⁻¹.

$$\text{BMR (kcal/day)} = 66.47 + (13.75 \times 90.9 \text{ kg}) + (5.0 \times 195.58 \text{ cm}) - (6.76 \times 27)$$

$$\text{BMR (kcal/day)} = (66.47 + 1249.87 + 977.9) - 182.5 = 2111.74 \text{ kcal/day}$$

$$\text{BMR (kcal/min)} = 2111.74 \text{ kcal/day} \times 1 \text{ day/24 hrs} \times 1 \text{ hr/60 min} = 1.466 \text{ kcal/min}$$

$$\text{BMR (L } O_2\text{/min)} = 1.466 \text{ kcal/min} \times 1 \text{ L } O_2\text{/5 kcals} = 0.293 \text{ L } O_2\text{/min}$$

$$\text{BMR (ml·kg⁻¹·min⁻¹)} = \frac{0.293 \text{ L } O_2\text{/min} \times 1000 \text{ ml/L } O_2}{90.9 \text{ kg}} = 3.23 \text{ ml·kg⁻¹·min⁻¹}$$

There are several practical reasons why dietitians and exercise professionals measure BMR or RMR. For instance, such measures can be used to determine total caloric needs for both healthy and diseased individuals; evaluate the chronic effects that various types of exercises have on resting metabolism; evaluate the chronic effects low-calorie diets have on resting metabolism; and screen for possible disease (e.g., cancer, endocrine abnormalities), since an unusually high or low resting metabolism is sometimes associated with disease.

Exercise Metabolic Rate

Exercise has a profound effect on the metabolic rate because various bodily systems (i.e., muscular, cardiorespiratory, nervous) require a considerable amount of energy (ATP) to sustain physical activity. Generally, light physical activity (walking) increases the metabolic rate 3–5 times above rest; moderate activity 6–10 times above rest, and vigorous to maximal activity 11–15 times above rest. Typical energy expenditure and oxygen cost values for physical activity are outlined in Table 10–2.

It is impractical to measure exercise metabolism with a whole-body calorimeter. Consequently, indirect measures based on oxygen consumption are utilized to determine caloric expenditure. In some situations, oxygen cost measures are also impractical due to the fact that expensive equipment and trained test technicians are required. Thus, prediction equations have been developed to estimate exercise metabolic rate.

Prediction of Exercise Metabolic Rate

The American College of Sports Medicine (ACSM) has developed prediction equations which, when properly used, can provide valid and reliable estimates of exercise oxygen cost or energy expenditure. Such equations are useful in that relatively accurate estimates of metabolic cost can be easily determined, both absolute and relative exercise intensity can be estimated for a variety of activities, and aerobic performance can be predicted (see Appendix D).

The ACSM metabolic formulae are essentially regression equations that predict directly measured oxygen cost or energy expenditure. As discussed in Chapter 1, all regression equations have the potential for making estimation errors. To minimize possible errors, the ACSM metabolic equations should be used as intended. For example,

1. The purpose of the equations is to relate exercise work rate to metabolic cost and vice versa.
2. Apply the formulae only to steady-state* aerobic exercise. An overestimation of actual oxygen cost will result if a high percentage of anaerobic energy is utilized during exercise. Such can occur in the initial minutes of exercise before a steady-state has been reached or when working above a steady-state (e.g., sprinting).
3. The formulae are designed for specific speeds and work rates. For instance, the walking equation should only be used for speeds between 50–100 $m \cdot min^{-1}$ (1.9–3.7 mph); the jogging equation only for speeds greater than 134 $m \cdot min^{-1}$ (> 5.0 mph); the cycle ergometer equation only for work rates between 300–1200 $kgm \cdot min^{-1}$; and the arm ergometry equation only for work rates between 150–750 $kgm \cdot min^{-1}$.
4. The jogging formulae apply to level and grade running on the treadmill and level running off the treadmill. Estimates for grade running off the treadmill should not be made because of increased prediction error.
5. The formulae cannot account for individual differences in exercise efficiency that may increase prediction error.
6. The formulae provide highest predictive accuracy when standard ergometric devices are used in a

*Steady-state exercise: The time period during which VO_2 remains at a constant (steady) value.

Table 10–2
Typical Energy Expenditure and Oxygen Cost for Exercise*

Exercise Intensity	kcal·min^{-1}	L O$_2$·min^{-1}	ml·kg^{-1}·min^{-1}	METS
Light	2.5–5	0.5–1.0	10–17	3–5
Moderate	5–10	1.0–2.0	20–35	6–10
Vigorous	12–20	2.5–4.0	40–50	11–15

*Approximate values for relatively fit college-aged individuals. Light intensity = walking; moderate intensity = slow jogging; vigorous intensity = running.

controlled environment. Running outdoors in extreme temperature, over a sandy or snowy terrain or in windy conditions, may greatly alter metabolic costs and increase predictive error. Also, equipment that is improperly calibrated or rail-holding during treadmill exercise can decrease predictive accuracy.

7. The equations are appropriate for adult men and women; however, predictions for children (<18 yr) should be avoided.

8. Accurate, reliable data should be entered into equations (e.g., actual walking speeds and grades) and errorless computations performed.

Research has demonstrated that, when properly applied, the ACSM formulae provide accurate estimates of metabolic cost and are suitable for a variety of non-laboratory applications. The ACSM equations consider three components of energy expenditure: the horizontal, vertical, and resting components. Calculations are expressed in units of VO_2 ($ml \cdot kg^{-1} \cdot min^{-1}$ or $ml \cdot min^{-1}$). The equivalent $1 \, L \, O_2 = 5$ kcal can be used to convert oxygen cost to energy expenditure (EE). The equivalent $1 \, mph = 26.82 \, m \cdot min^{-1}$ can be used to obtain desirable speed units (Table 10–3). Note that these prediction equations provide estimates of exercise oxygen consumption that are corrected to STPD. (See Chapter 12 and Appendix C for more information about STPD correction factors.) Common equivalents used in metabolic computations are provided in Table 10–4.

Table 10–3
Treadmill Speed Conversions*

mph	$m \cdot min^{-1}$	mph	$m \cdot min^{-1}$
2.0	53.6	7.0	187.7
2.5	67.0	7.5	201.1
3.0	80.5	8.0	214.6
3.5	93.9	8.5	228.0
4.0	107.3	9.0	241.4
4.5	120.7	9.5	254.8
5.0	134.1	10.0	268.2
5.5	147.5	10.5	281.6
6.0	160.9	11.0	295.0
6.5	174.3	11.5	308.4

*Based on $1 \, mph = 26.82 \, m \cdot min^{-1}$

Walking equation:

$$VO_2 \, (ml \cdot kg^{-1} \cdot min^{-1}) = [speed \, (m \cdot min^{-1})$$
$$\times \, 0.1 \, \frac{ml \cdot kg^{-1} \cdot min^{-1}}{m \cdot min^{-1}} \,]$$
$$+ \, [grade \times speed \, (m \cdot min^{-1})$$
$$\times \, 1.8 \, \frac{ml \cdot kg^{-1} \cdot min^{-1}}{m \cdot min^{-1}} \,]$$
$$+ \, [3.5 \, ml \cdot kg^{-1} \cdot min^{-1}]$$

Computation examples: What are the estimated oxygen cost and energy expenditure (EE) of a 3.5 mph level-grade walk? Assume a body mass of 82 kg.

$$VO_2 = [93.8 \, m \cdot min^{-1} \times 0.1 \, \frac{ml \cdot kg^{-1} \cdot min^{-1}}{m \cdot min^{-1}} \,]$$
$$+ \, [0 \times 93.8 \, m \cdot min^{-1} \times 1.8 \, \frac{ml \cdot kg^{-1} \cdot min^{-1}}{m \cdot min^{-1}} \,]$$
$$+ \, [3.5 \, ml \cdot kg^{-1} \cdot min^{-1}] = 12.88 \, ml \cdot kg^{-1} \cdot min^{-1}$$
$$EE = 12.8 \, ml \cdot kg^{-1} \cdot min^{-1} \times 82 \, kg = 1049.6 \, ml \cdot min^{-1}$$
$$\text{or } 1.049 \, L \cdot min^{-1}$$
$$1.049 \, L \cdot min^{-1} \times 5 \, kcal \cdot L^{-1} = 5.24 \, kcal \cdot min^{-1}$$

Jogging equation (treadmill):

$$VO_2 \, (ml \cdot kg^{-1} \cdot min^{-1}) = [speed \, (m \cdot min^{-1})$$
$$\times \, 0.2 \, \frac{ml \cdot kg^{-1} \cdot min^{-1}}{m \cdot min^{-1}} \,]$$
$$+ \, [grade \times speed \, (m \cdot min^{-1})$$
$$\times \, 1.8 \, \frac{ml \cdot kg^{-1} \cdot min^{-1}}{m \cdot min^{-1}} \times 0.5]$$
$$+ \, [3.5 \, ml \cdot kg^{-1} \cdot min^{-1}]$$

Note: For non-treadmill application, use the same equation but exclude 0.5 from the grade portion of the formula.

Computation example: What are the estimated oxygen cost and energy expenditure (EE) of a 5.5 mph 10% grade treadmill jog? Assume a body mass of 77 kg.

$$VO_2 = [147.5 \, m \cdot min^{-1} \times 0.2 \, \frac{ml \cdot kg^{-1} \cdot min^{-1}}{m \cdot min^{-1}} \,] +$$

Table 10–4
Conversions and Useful Relationships

Parameter	Common Units	Conversion Factors
Time	second (sec) minute (min) hour (hr) day (d) week (wk) month (mo)	60 sec = 1 min 60 min = 1 hr 1 d = 24 hr = 1440 min 1 wk = 7 d = 10,080 min
Distance	centimeter (cm) meter (m)* kilometer (km) inch (in) foot (ft) mile (mi)	100 cm = 1 m 1 m = 39.37 in = 3.28 ft 1 in = 2.54 cm 1 mi = 5280 ft = 1.6 km 1 km = 0.625 mi
Mass or Weight	pounds (lb) kilogram (kg)*	1 lb = 0.4536 kg 1 kg = 2.204 lbs
Force	kilopond (kp) Newton (N)*	1 kg ≈ 1 kp = 9.8 Newton
Speed	miles per hour (mph) meters per minute (m/min)* kilometer per hour (km/hr)	1 mph = 26.82 m/min 1m/min = 0.0373 mph 1 km/hr = 16 m/min 1 mph = 1.609 km/hr
Work	kilojoule (kJ)* kilogram meter (kg·m)	1 kJ = 0.2381 kcal
Power or Work rate	watt (W)* kilogram meter per minute (kg·m/min)	1 watt = 6.12 kg·m/min
Energy Expenditure or Oxygen Uptake	kilojoule (kJ)* kilocalories per minute (kcal/min) milliliters O_2 per (ml/min) liters O_2 per minute (L/min) milliliters O_2 per kilogram body mass per minute (ml·kg^{-1}·min^{-1})	1 kJ = 0.2381 kcal 5 kcal = 1 LO_2 1 kcal/min = 69.78 W 1 kcal/min = 426.4 kgm/min 1000 ml/min = 1 L/min 1 MET = 3.5 ml·kg^{-1}·min^{-1}

*Preferred SI units

$$[0.10 \times 147.5 \text{ m·min}^{-1} \times 1.8 \ \frac{\text{ml·kg}^{-1}\cdot\text{min}^{-1}}{\text{m·min}^{-1}}$$

$$\times 0.5] + [3.5 \text{ ml·kg}^{-1}\cdot\text{min}^{-1}] =$$

$$29.5 + 13.27 + 3.5 = 46.27 \text{ ml·kg}^{-1}\cdot\text{min}^{-1}$$

$$EE = 46.27 \text{ ml·kg}^{-1}\cdot\text{min}^{-1} \times 77 \text{ kg} = 3562.7 \text{ ml·min}^{-1}$$

$$\text{or } 3.562 \text{ L·min}^{-1}$$

$$3.562 \text{ L·min}^{-1} \times 5 \text{ kcal·L}^{-1} = 17.81 \text{ kcal·min}^{-1}$$

Note: The grade should be input in decimal form and not as a percent.

Leg cycle ergometry equation:

$$VO_2 \text{ (ml·min}^{-1}) = [\text{work rate (kgm·min}^{-1}) \times 2\frac{\text{ml}}{\text{kgm}}]$$

$$+ [3.5 \text{ ml·kg}^{-1}\cdot\text{min}^{-1} \times \text{body mass (kg)}]$$

Computation example: What are the estimated oxygen cost and energy expenditure for leg cycle ergometry when pedaling at a work rate of 750 kgm·min⁻¹? Assume a body mass of 80 kg.

$$VO_2 = [750 \text{ kgm·min}^{-1}) \times 2 \frac{ml}{kgm}] +$$

$$[3.5 \text{ ml·kg}^{-1}\text{·min}^{-1} \times 80 \text{ kg}] = 1780 \text{ ml·min}^{-1}$$

or $1780 \text{ ml·min}^{-1} \div 80 \text{ kg} = 22.3 \text{ ml·kg}^{-1}\text{·min}^{-1}$

$$EE = 1780 \text{ ml·min}^{-1} = 1.78 \text{ L·min}^{-1}$$

$$1.78 \text{ L·min}^{-1} \times 5 \text{ kcal·L}^{-1} = 8.9 \text{ kcal·min}^{-1}$$

Stepping equation:

$$VO_2 \text{ (ml·kg}^{-1}\text{·min}^{-1}) = [\text{steps·min}^{-1}$$

$$\times 0.35 \frac{ml \cdot kg^{-1} \cdot min^{-1}}{steps \cdot min^{-1}}]$$

$$+ [m\text{·step}^{-1} \times \text{steps·min}^{-1} \times 1.33$$

$$\times 1.8 \frac{ml \cdot kg^{-1} \cdot min^{-1}}{m \cdot min^{-1}}]$$

Computation examples: What are the estimated oxygen cost and energy expenditure (EE) of stepping at a rate of 20 steps/min? Assume a step height of 0.20 meters and a body mass of 69 kg.

$$VO_2 = [20 \text{ steps·min}^{-1} \times 0.35 \frac{ml \cdot kg^{-1} \cdot min^{-1}}{steps \cdot min^{-1}}] +$$

$$[0.20 \text{ m·step} \times 20 \text{ steps·min} \times 1.33$$

$$\times 1.8 \frac{ml \cdot kg^{-1} \cdot min^{-1}}{m \cdot min^{-1}}] =$$

$$7 + 9.576 = 16.57 \text{ ml·kg}^{-1}\text{·min}^{-1}$$

$$EE = 16.57 \text{ ml·kg}^{-1}\text{·min}^{-1} \times 69 \text{ kg} = 1143.7 \text{ ml·min}^{-1}$$

$$\text{or } 1.143 \text{ L·min}^{-1}$$

$$1.143 \text{ L·min}^{-1} \times 5 \text{ kcal·L}^{-1} = 5.71 \text{ kcal·min}^{-1}$$

Arm Ergometry equation:

$$VO_2 \text{ (ml·min}^{-1}) = [\text{work rate (kgm·min}^{-1}) \times 3.0 \frac{ml}{kgm}]$$

$$+ [3.5 \text{ ml·kg}^{-1}\text{·min}^{-1} \times \text{body mass (kg)}]$$

Computation examples: What are the estimated oxygen cost and energy expenditure (EE) for arm ergometry with a work rate of 450 kgm·min⁻¹ and a body mass of 95 kg?

$$VO_2 = [450 \text{ kgm·min}^{-1} \times 3.0 \frac{ml}{kgm}] +$$

$$[3.5 \text{ ml·kg}^{-1}\text{·min}^{-1} \times 95 \text{ kg}] =$$

$$1350 + 332.5 = 1682.5 \text{ ml·min}^{-1}$$

or $1682.5 \text{ ml·min}^{-1} \div 95 \text{ kg} = 17.7 \text{ ml·kg}^{-1}\text{·min}^{-1}$

$$EE = 1682.5 \text{ ml·min}^{-1} = 1.68 \text{ L·min}^{-1}$$

$$1.68 \text{ L·min}^{-1} \times 5 \text{ kcal·L}^{-1} = 8.4 \text{ kcal·min}^{-1}$$

An understanding of the metabolic cost of various exercises allows one to prescribe a safe and effective exercise intensity for individuals of differing ability; to compute estimates of weekly physical activity energy expenditure and the likely risk for various diseases; and to compute total energy costs to better plan daily dietary needs.

SELECTED REFERENCES

Adams, G. M. (1990). *Exercise Physiology Lab Manual.* Dubuque, Iowa: Wm. C. Brown Publishers, pp: 252.

Adams, W. C. (1967). Influence of age, sex, and body weight on the energy expenditure of bicycle riding. *J. Appl. Physiol.* 22:539–545.

American College of Sports Medicine (ACSM). (1991). *Guidelines of Exercise Testing and Prescription* (4th edition). Philadelphia: Lea & Febiger, pp: 285–300.

Dill, D. B. (1965). Oxygen used in horizontal and grade walking and running on the treadmill. *J. Appl. Physiol.* 20:19–22.

Harris, J. A., and F. G. Benedict (1919). A biometric study of basal metabolism in man. Washington, D.C.: Carnegie Institution of Washington (publication 279).

Heyward, V. H. (1991). *Advanced Fitness Assessment and Exercise Prescription.* Champaign, Illinois: Human Kinetics, pp: 33–36.

STATION 1
Basal/Resting Metabolic Rate

Research Questions

1. What is the difference between observed RMR (kcal/min) and estimated BMR (kcal/min)? Is the predicted score within ± 10% of the observed score? Provide plausible reasons for any differences between predicted and observed scores.

2. Basal metabolic rate has been shown to decrease 20–30% as a result of a very-low-calorie diet (i.e., 400–700 kcal/day). If your own predicted BMR were to decrease by 30%, how many kcals would not be expended per year as a result of this decrease in BMR? Discuss implications.

Data Collection

Your instructor will administer the test for RMR measurement and may ask for your assistance. Record the test data provided by your instructor on Chart 10–1. Also compute the necessary calculations and record on Chart 10–1.

Measurement Of Metabolic Rate
Assignment

STATION 1

Chart 10–1 Comparison of Predicted and Observed VO$_2$			
Parameter	*Predicted VO$_2$* *ml·kg^{-1}·min^{-1}*	*Observed VO$_2$* *ml·kg^{-1}·min^{-1}*	*Difference*
Resting			
Walk: 3.0 mph, 7.5% grade			
Jog: 6.0 mph, level grade			
Cycle: 600 kgm·min^{-1}			

Research Conclusions

Show work for all computations. Express oxygen cost in ml·kg^{-1}·min^{-1}.

1. What is the difference between observed RMR (kcal/min) and estimated BMR (kcal/min)? Is the predicted score within ± 10% of the observed score? Record results on Chart 10–1. Provide plausible reasons for any differences between predicted and observed scores.

2. Basal metabolic rate has been shown to decrease 20–30% as a result of a very-low-calorie diet (i.e., 400–700 kcal/day). If your own predicted BMR were to decrease by 30%, how many kcals would not be expended per year as a result of this decrease in BMR? Discuss implications.

STATION 2
. . . .
Exercise Metabolic Rate

Research Questions

1. What is the difference between observed and estimated oxygen cost for a treadmill walk of 3.0 mph and 7.5 % grade?

2. What is the difference between observed and estimated oxygen cost for a treadmill jog of 6.0 mph and level grade?

3. What is the difference between observed and estimated oxygen cost when pedaling on a leg cycle ergometer at a work rate of 600 kgm·min^{-1}? (Use the body mass of the subject to convert from ml·min^{-1} to ml·kg^{-1}·min^{-1}.)

4. Prioritize the accuracy of the VO$_2$ predictions for the walk, jog, and cycle (Chart 10–1). Were all predictions within ± 5 ml·kg^{-1}·min^{-1} of the observed score? Provide plausible reasons for any differences between predicted and observed scores and modes of exercise.

5. What is the estimated oxygen cost (ml·kg^{-1}·min^{-1}) and energy expenditure (kcal·min^{-1}) of jogging a marathon (26.2 miles) in 3 hours? Assume the marathon runner has a body mass of 65 kg. Show work. Provide at least three reasons why such an estimate may be in error.

Data Collection

Your instructor will administer the tests necessary to determine observed exercise metabolic rate. You should assist your instructor as needed. Record the test data provided by your instructor on Chart 10–1. Show your work for the necessary calculations and record on Chart 10–1.

Name: _____ Date: _____

Exercise Metabolic Rate
Assignment

Research Conclusions

Show work for all your computations. Express oxygen cost in $ml \cdot kg^{-1} \cdot min^{-1}$.

1. What is the difference between observed and estimated oxygen costs for a treadmill walk of 3.0 mph and 7.5 % grade? Record results on Chart 10–1.

2. What is the difference between observed and estimated oxygen costs for a treadmill jog of 6.0 mph and level grade? Record results on Chart 10–1.

3. What is the difference between observed and estimated oxygen cost when pedaling on a leg cycle ergometer at a work rate of 600 $kgm \cdot min^{-1}$? Use the body mass of the subject to convert from $ml \cdot min^{-1}$ to $ml \cdot kg^{-1} \cdot min^{-1}$. Show work. Record results on Chart 10–1.

4. Prioritize the accuracy of the VO$_2$ predictions for the walk, jog, and cycle (Chart 10–1). Were all predictions within $\pm$ 5 ml·kg^{-1}·min^{-1} of the observed score? Provide plausible reasons for any differences between predicted and observed scores and modes of exercise.

5. What is the estimated oxygen cost (ml·kg^{-1}·min^{-1}) and energy expenditure (kcal·min^{-1}) of jogging a marathon (26.2 miles) in 3 hours? Assume the marathon runner has a body mass of 65 kg. Show work. Provide at least three reasons why such an estimate may be in error.

Name:_____ Date: _____

Describe several ways the information learned in this lab can be applied to your chosen field of interest and/or your personal life. Be specific and provide practical examples.

Name: _____   Date: _____

11

Resting and Exercise Electrocardiograms
. . . .
Pre-Laboratory Assignment

1. Describe at least two purposes for ECG measurements.

2. Draw a typical ECG tracing and label all basic components.

3. Explain what should be done to prepare the electrode site for ECG measurements.

4. If there are 10 mm between two successive R waves, what would be the computed heart rate? Does this appear to be a resting or exercise heart rate, based on your results? Show work. (Assume a standard chart speed of 25 mm/sec.)

5. ❑ Check the box if you have read each research question for this lab and are familiar with the data collection procedures regarding each research question.

11
Resting And Exercise Electrocardiograms

Each time the myocardium contracts and relaxes, a small electrical current is conducted through the body. An electrocardiograph is designed to measure this electrical current and provide an electrocardiogram (ECG)—a graphical tracing of cardiac muscle activity. Cardiologists are trained to interpret ECG tracings and can use this information to detect possible structural and functional abnormalities within the myocardium.

The conduction system within the heart consists of several components. The sino-atrial (SA) node is located on the posterior wall of the right atrium near the opening of the superior vena cava. The internodal pathways collectively merge upon the atrioventricular (AV) node, which is located in the right posterior portion of the interatrial septum. The AV node and Bundle of His propagate the impulse across the atrioventricular junction. The Bundle of His divides into the Left and Right Bundle Branches (LBB and RBB), which carry the electrical impulse to the left and right ventricles, respectively. The terminal endings of the bundle branches are the Purkinje fibers, which extend into the endocardium (Figure 11–1).

A normal conduction cycle of the heart originates in the SA node and spreads throughout the internodal pathways and atria to the AV node. The AV node imposes a slight delay (about 0.1 seconds) to allow the atria to contract and allow the ventricles to fill. The slight delay also protects the ventricles from conduction problems within the atria (i.e., atrial flutter or fibrillation). Action potentials enter the ventricles by way of the Bundle of His, dividing into the left and right bundle branches, which terminate as Purkinje fibers in the endocardium. As depolarization of the atria and ventricles is completed, repolarization of myocardium follows.

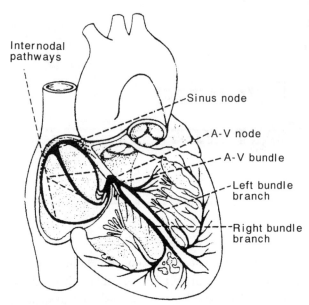

Internodal pathways

Sinus node

A-V node

A-V bundle

Left bundle branch

Right bundle branch

Figure 11–1

There are three basic components of the ECG tracing (Figure 11–1): the P wave, representing atrial depolarization; the QRS complex, representing ventricular depolarization; and the T wave, representing ventricular repolarization. (Note: Atrial repolarization is normally hidden by the large QRS complex and therefore does not appear on the ECG tracing.)

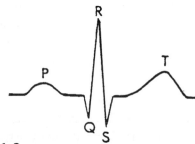

Figure 11–2

The 12-lead ECG is a set of 12 different views of the heart as depicted by individual electrodes or a combination of electrodes. The configuration of the ECG recording will appear different in each of the 12 leads since each electrode views the activities of the heart from a slightly different position. Note that even though there are only 10 electrodes used, there are actually 12 leads or views that can be generated for examination.

Subject Preparation

The quality of the ECG often depends on subject preparation and electrode placement. The quality of ECG recordings is improved as interference with re-

cordings is reduced. Interference can be diminished when body oil, soil, and hair are removed from the skin prior to ECG measurement.

Clothing: It is important to wear appropriate clothing for a resting or exercise ECG. Men are asked to remove their shirts and women are asked to wear loose-fitting button-down blouses or hospital gowns.

Volunteer: The volunteer should be lying down in a supine position. Throughout the ECG measurement, inform your subject of the procedures you are about to perform and why such procedures are necessary.

Type of Electrode: For resting ECG measurements, either self-adhering electrodes or strap and suction-cup-mounted electrodes may be used; however, to reduce costs, many labs use strap and suction-cup-mounted electrodes. For exercise ECG measurements, only the pre-packaged, self-adhering electrodes should be used.

Electrode Sites: The anatomical sites for the ten electrodes are described below:

Limb Leads: When strap-mounted electrodes are used, place limb leads superior to and on the ventral side of the wrists and along the medial side of the ankles (Figure 11–3). When self-adhering electrodes are used, position them just below the midline of the clavicles and on the lower ribs (Figure 11–4).

Chest Leads: Chest lead locations are the same for both self-adhering and suction-cup electrodes.

V_1—fourth intercostal space to the right of the sternum

V_2—fourth intercostal space to the left of the sternum

V_3—midway between V_2 and V_4

V_4—left mid-clavicular line on fifth intercostal space

V_5—left anterior axillary line at same level as V_4

V_6—left mid-axillary line at same level as V_4 and V_5

Electrode Preparation: All hair, lotions, soil, and body oils must be removed from the electrode site. To do this, locate the electrode site; shave any body hair

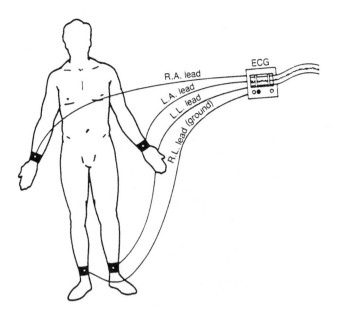

Figure 11–3

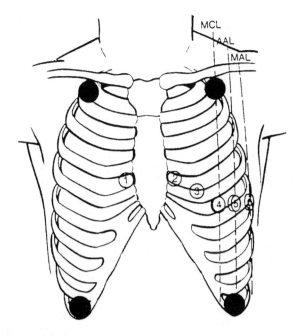

Figure 11–4

from the landmark with a clean, dry disposable razor; gently rub the landmark with a small piece of fine-grain sandpaper; and wipe the area clean with a cotton swab saturated with rubbing alcohol (this may sting the subject a little). The skin color at the electrode site should be slightly red at this point. Be sure not to touch the electrode site with your fingers after it has been prepared. To prevent the possible spread of disease, the razor, sandpaper, and alcohol swab must be discarded after a single use.

When strap-mounted or suction-cup electrodes are used, first apply a small amount of electrode gel to the landmark; then place the limb electrodes over the landmark and strap them securely to the limb. Be careful not to attach the straps too tightly.

Connect the ECG cables to the limb electrodes as follows:

Right Arm (RA, white): connect to the right arm
Left Arm (LA, black): connect to the left arm
Left Leg (LL, red): connect to the left leg
Right Leg (RL, green): connect to the right leg

When suction electrodes are used for chest leads, attach the cables to the suction cups prior to placement on the chest. Apply a small amount of electrode gel at each chest landmark. Squeeze each suction cup and position it on the appropriate chest electrode site.

When self-adhering electrodes are used for chest leads, peel off the protective backing and apply at the appropriate chest electrode site. Press the electrode firmly onto the skin. Snap the cables onto the proper chest electrodes. (Note that no electrode gel is needed when self-adhering electrodes are used.)

ECG Measurement

1. Calibrate the ECG machine.
2. Double check all cables to make sure they are attached to the correct electrode.
3. Record a tracing for each of the 12 ECG leads by pressing the appropriate control buttons on the ECG machine.
4. Label each ECG tracing (i.e., date, subject's name and age; subject body position—supine or standing—and whether it is a resting or exercise ECG).

Note: If all electrode connections are made correctly, the stylus pen will move smoothly in response to each heart beat. If the pens are erratic and have visible measurement "noise," recheck the cable connections and electrode attachments. When all leads are erratic, check the green right leg lead (ground). Standard 12-lead ECG tracings should appear as illustrated in Figure 11–5.

Heart Rate Measurement

To determine heart rate from an ECG recording, it is essential to know that the duration of time between two successive vertical lines (1 mm) on standard ECG

RESTING AND EXERCISE ELECTROCARDIOGRAMS

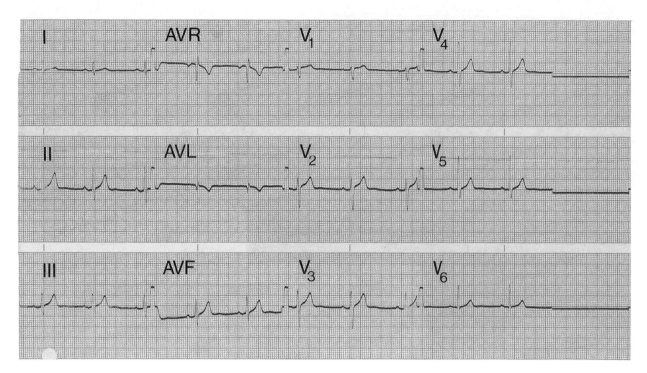

Figure 11–5

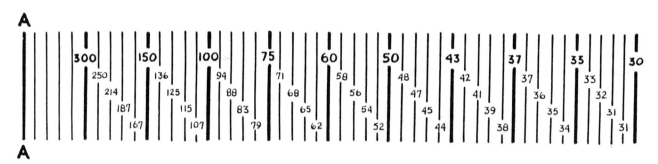

Figure 11–6

paper represents 0.04 seconds at a paper speed of 25 mm/sec (Figure 11–5).

There are three methods that can be used to determine heart rate from an ECG tracing:

Method 1: Count the number of cardiac cycles in a one-minute ECG recording. The initial QRS complex should be counted as zero and is considered the reference point for the 1-minute time period.

This method is appropriate when there are rhythm irregularities in the ECG measurement, but uses a great deal of ECG paper. When heart rates appear regular (each heart beat is separated by an equal time period), then methods 2 or 3 are recommended.

Method 2: Calculate heart rate based on the duration of time between beats. Count the number of 1 mm squares between consecutive R waves. Divide this number into 1500 (at a paper speed of 25 mm/sec, there are 1500 mm/min). For example, if there are 15 mm between an R–R interval, then

$$HR = 1500 \div 15 = 100 \text{ bpm}$$

An alternative eyeball approach is to use the aid outlined in Figure 11–6, which is simply an extension of the formula above. For example, find two consecutive R waves (consider the first R wave at the A position) and count the heavy lines between them. If there are 2 heavy lines between the R waves (10 mm) this would equal a heart rate of 150 bpm. Oftentimes the R waves won't match up exactly on the bold lines, but still this method can provide a quick approximation of heart rate, especially if you memorize and apply the numbers 300, 150, 100, 75, and 60 (Figure 11–6). Thus, if there were between 2 and 3 bold lines between R waves, you would know the heart rate was between 100 and 150 bpm; likewise, if there were between 4 and 5 bold lines between R waves, you would know the heart rate was somewhere between 60 and 75 bpm. Of course, for greater accuracy you could use the formula above or methods 1 and 3.

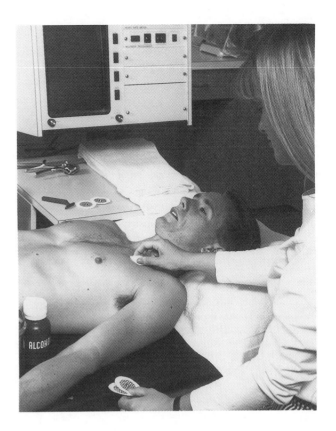

Method 3: Calculate heart rate from 3- or 6-second intervals. Most ECG paper has 3-second marks on the top border of the paper. Count the number of cardiac cycles in a 3- or 6-second time period. Multiply the number of cycles by 20 or 10, respectively, to determine heart rate. For example, if there are 5½ complete cardiac cycles in a 3-second period, then

$$HR = 5\tfrac{1}{2} \times 20 = 110 \text{ bpm}$$

Research Questions

1. What were the beats-per-minute difference between the supine and standing ECG heart rate measurements for your volunteer? Describe at least two reasons why standing heart rate may be higher than supine heart rate.
2. Do heart rate measurement methods 2 and 3 generate an exercise heart rate within ± 5 bpm of each other? Provide possible reasons for any differences.
3. Describe how heart rate measurement methods 2 and 3 could be modified to improve their accuracy.
4. Determine specific differences between resting and exercise P-waves, QRS-complexes, and T-waves. Quantify all your observations in millimeters (mm). Provide possible reasons for any differences.
5. Determine the difference in time (sec) between resting and exercise ECG tracings. Evaluate differences from a) the initiation of the P-wave to the termination of the T-wave and b) from the termination of the T-wave to the initiation of the P-wave. Discuss your findings.

Data Collection

1. Prepare the subject for a 12-lead ECG tracing by prepping the 10 electrode sites discussed above. Attach the cables to the appropriate electrode.
2. Calibrate the ECG machine with the help of your instructor.
3. Record a supine and standing tracing for each of the 12 ECG leads.
4. Have your subject walk on a treadmill or ride a stationary bicycle for several minutes at a moderate intensity. Record an ECG tracing during exercise.
5. Label each ECG tracing (i.e., date, subject's name and age; subject body position—supine or standing—and whether it is a resting or exercise ECG).
6. Photocopy the ECG tracings for each class member.
7. Mount two ECG tracings for both supine and standing positions and determine the heart rate for each. Record information on Chart 11–1.

8. Mount an exercise ECG tracing and determine the heart rate with methods 2 and 3. Record information on Chart 11–2.

SELECTED REFERENCES

Adams, G. M. (1990). *Exercise Physiology Lab Manual*. Dubuque, Iowa: Wm. C. Brown Publishers, pp: 135–142.

Dubin, D. (1974). *Rapid Interpretation of EKG's* (3rd edition). Tampa, Florida: Cover Publishing Co.

Fisher, A. G., and C. R. Jensen (1990). *Scientific Basis of Athletic Conditioning* (3rd edition). Philadelphia: Lea & Febiger, pp: 77–83.

Fox, E. L., R. W. Bowers, and M. L. Foss (1988). *The Physiological Basis of Physical Education and Athletics* (4th edition). Philadelphia: Saunders College Publishing, pp: 245–248.

Grauer, K. and Curry, R.W., Jr. (1992). *Clinical Electrocardiography*. Boston: Blackwell Scientific Publications.

Marriot, J. L. (1987). *ECG / PDQ*. Baltimore: Williams and Wilkins.

McArdle, W. D., F. I. Katch, and V. L. Katch (1991). *Exercise Physiology: Energy, Nutrition, and Human Performance* (3rd edition). Philadelphia: Lea & Febiger, pp: 313–316, 723–726.

Powers, S. K., and E. T. Howley (1990). *Exercise Physiology: Theory and Application to Fitness and Performance*. Dubuque, Iowa: Wm. C. Brown Publishers, pp: 180–184.

Resting and Exercise Electrocardiograms
Assignment

Chart 11–1
Resting ECG Data Sheet

Name: _____   Date: _____

Age: _____   ☐ Male   ☐ Female

Supine ECG: Paste two supine ECG tracings in the space provided below. Record the lead and heart rate in the spaces provided. Show heart rate computations.

Lead _____   Lead _____

Heart Rate: _____ bpm   Heart Rate: _____ bpm

Standing ECG: Paste two standing ECG tracings in the space provided below. Record the lead and heart rate in the spaces provided. Show heart rate computations.

Lead _____   Lead _____

Heart Rate: _____ bpm   Heart Rate: _____ bpm

Chart 11–2
Exercise ECG Data Sheet

Name: _____   Date: _____

Age: _____

☐ Male   ☐ Treadmill

☐ Female   ☐ Bicycle

                          ☐ Other

Exercise ECG: Paste an exercise ECG tracing in the space provided below. Record the lead and heart rates in the spaces provided. Show heart rate computations.

Heart Rate via ECG tracing:

Lead: _____

Method 2: _____ bpm

Method 3: _____ bpm

Difference: _____ bpm

Research Conclusions

1. What were the beats-per-minute difference between the supine and standing ECG heart rate measurements for your volunteer? Describe at least two reasons why standing heart rate may be higher than supine heart rate.

2. Do heart rate measurement methods 2 and 3 generate an exercise heart rate within ±5 bpm of each other? Provide possible reasons for any differences.

3. Describe how heart rate measurement methods 2 and 3 could be modified to improve their accuracy.

4. Determine specific differences between resting and exercise P-waves, QRS-complexes, and T-waves. Quantify all your observations in millimeters (mm). Provide possible reasons for any differences.

5. Determine the difference in time (sec) between resting and exercise ECG tracings. Evaluate differences from a) the initiation of the P-wave to the termination of the T-wave and b) from the termination of the T-wave to the initiation of the P-wave. Discuss your findings.

Name: _____ Date: _____

. . . .
Lab 11 Summary

Describe several ways the information learned in this lab can be applied to your chosen field of interest and/or your personal life. Be specific and provide practical examples.

12
Measurement of VO$_{2max}$
. . . .
Pre-Laboratory Assignment

1. Describe at least three important characteristics of a maximal graded exercise test.

2. List the criteria used to determine whether or not a VO$_{2max}$ test is valid.

3. Describe the meaning of the term "MET". What would be the maximum MET score of a female athlete who has a VO$_{2max}$ of 49.3 ml·kg^{-1}·min^{-1}? Show your work.

4. What does RER stand for, and how is it computed? Why should an RER be computed during a VO_{2max} test?

5. What does RPE stand for? Describe the objective of RPE scores. What does an RPE of 13 indicate?

6. ☐ Check the box if you have read each research question and are familiar with the data collection procedures regarding each research question.

12

Measurement Of VO$_{2max}$

PURPOSE

The purpose of this lab is to help you understand how to measure maximal oxygen uptake (VO$_{2max}$) using computer-assisted techniques.

STUDENT LEARNING OBJECTIVES

1. Understand how to administer a maximal exertion test designed to measure VO$_{2max}$.
2. Be able to interpret the results of a VO$_{2max}$ test.

NECESSARY EQUIPMENT

Motor-driven treadmill or bicycle ergometer
Gas analysis equipment
Ventilation measurement equipment
VO$_{2max}$ computer software
Blood pressure equipment
Heart rate monitoring device (ECG, telemetry)
Mouthpiece and nose clips

In recent years, improved technology has provided better, faster, and easier methods to measure and evaluate VO$_{2max}$. The information that years ago required hours to compute can now be generated in a matter of seconds. Accordingly, computerized systems allow exercise scientists to collect a variety of meaningful information during both rest and physical activity.

Graded exercise tests can be designed to measure VO$_{2max}$ or functional capacity. Such tests should require a minimum duration of about 6–10 minutes; involve a mode of exercise that utilizes large skeletal muscles (e.g., walking, jogging, cycling); and cause participants to put forth maximum effort. Several quantifiable criteria are used to determine whether or not a VO$_{2max}$ test is considered valid (Table 12–1).

When the criteria in Table 12–1 are not satisfied during a maximal exertion exercise test, then the measurement is termed VO$_{2peak}$. This implies that the highest VO$_2$ value was recorded, but it was not necessarily a maximal value. VO$_{2peak}$ measures are common when individuals walk on a treadmill up a steep grade, and their calf muscles become fatigued. Thus, the individual terminates the test because of lower leg pain and

Table 12–1
Criteria for VO$_{2max}$*

1. Exercise heart rate no more than 15 bpm below age-predicted maximum heart rate (HR$_{max}$ = 220 – age)
2. Respiratory exchange ratio (RER) ≥ 1.1
3. Oxygen consumption levels off despite an increase in work*

* At least two of the above three criteria must be achieved before a VO$_{2max}$ can be considered at a maximum level of exertion.
Source: Kline (1987).

not because he or she has reached a maximal level of exertion. To circumvent this problem, a faster treadmill speed and lower grade are recommended for the VO_{2max} test (especially for younger, relatively fit populations). VO_{2peak} measures are also common when individuals are not motivated to put forth maximum effort and terminate the test prematurely.

A variety of physiological responses are often evaluated during a VO_{2max} test. These include heart rate, blood pressure, symptoms, respiratory exchange ratio (RER), and rating of perceived exertion (RPE). The evaluation of such information can be used to help ensure the safety of exercise tests, ascertain subjects' relative exercise intensity, and determine whether or not physiological responses to the VO_{2max} are normal.

Heart rate can be measured with telemetry equipment or an electrocardiograph. The advantage of using the electrocardiograph is that additional information about the normality of cardiac function during exercise is provided. Electrocardiographs are often used by physicians to screen for coronary heart disease; however, such equipment can also be used to measure heart rate.

Blood pressure can be measured during exercise when bodily movement of the subject does not impede the measurement process. It is relatively easy to measure blood pressure during treadmill walking and cycle ergometry; however, treadmill jogging greatly hinders the ability to obtain accurate blood pressure measures.

A variety of symptoms should be monitored during and immediately following maximal exertion exercise. These include: dyspnea (labored breathing), fatigue, angina (chest pain), ataxia (failure of muscular coordination), nausea, or pallor (paleness). Some symptoms are observable, while others must be communicated by the participant.

A respiratory exchange ratio (RER) should be computed (via computer) during a VO_{2max} test. An RER is equal to the volume of carbon dioxide expired per minute divided by the volume of oxygen consumed per minute. RER values reflect the type of fuel (i.e., carbohydrate, fat) utilized during rest and exercise. As RER values increase, a higher proportion of carbohydrate is utilized compared to fat (Table 12–2). An important criterion for a VO_{2max} test is a RER ≥ 1.1 (Table 12–1), since a high RER generally reflects that a subject has reached a maximal level of exertion.

Table 12–2
RER Values and Substrate Metabolism

RER	kcal/L O_2	Percent of Total kcal by	
		Carbohydrates	Fat
0.70	4.68	0.0	100.00
0.72	4.70	4.4	95.6
0.74	4.73	11.3	88.7
0.76	4.75	18.1	81.9
0.78	4.77	24.9	75.1
0.80	4.80	31.7	68.3
0.82	4.82	38.6	61.4
0.84	4.85	45.4	54.6
0.86	4.88	52.2	47.8
0.88	4.90	59.0	41.0
0.90	4.92	65.9	34.1
0.92	4.95	72.7	27.3
0.94	4.97	79.5	20.5
0.96	5.00	86.3	13.7
0.98	5.02	93.2	6.8
1.00	5.05	100.0	0.0

Ratings of perceived exertion (RPEs) are used to quantify participants' feelings and sensations regarding the stress of physical activity. Subjective measures of exertion are useful since they can be compared to physiological measures (e.g., heart rate) and provide additional information about the intensity of exercise. A number of studies have indicated that RPE scores are strongly correlated to objective measures of exercise intensity. The Borg 15-point RPE scale, illustrated in Table 12–3, is frequently used during a VO_{2max} test to ascertain perceived exertion values.

VO_2 Calculations

The various principles and equations used to compute VO_2 range from simple to complex. In simplistic terms, VO_2 equals the volume of oxygen inspired (per minute) minus the volume of oxygen expired (per minute). This implies that the oxygen that enters the lungs but doesn't come back out is taken in by the body (consumed) to facilitate aerobic energy production. A formula to represent this principle would be:

Table 12–3
RPE Scale

6	
7	Very Very Light
8	
9	Very Light
10	
11	Fairly Light
12	
13	Somewhat Hard
14	
15	Hard
16	
17	Very Hard
18	
19	Very Very Hard
20	

Source: Borg (1970).

$$VO_2 = V_IO_2 - V_EO_2$$

Where:
VO_2 = volume of oxygen consumed per minute
V_IO_2 = volume of inspired oxygen per minute
V_EO_2 = volume of expired oxygen per minute

Computation example: What would be the VO_2 (oxygen consumption) for a marathon runner who inspires 20.7 L of O_2 per minute and expires 16.0 L of O_2 per minute?

$$VO_2 = 20.7 \text{ L } O_2/\text{min} - 16.0 \text{ L } O_2/\text{min}$$
$$= 4.7 \text{ L } O_2/\text{min}$$

To determine V_IO_2, the volume of inspired air per minute is multiplied by the fraction of oxygen in the atmosphere. Likewise to determine V_EO_2, the volume of expired air per minute is multiplied by the fraction of expired air composed of oxygen. Metabolic gas analyzers can be utilized to determine the concentration of gas in ventilated air and an air meter (electronic pneumotachometer) can be used to quantify the volume of ventilated air. Thus, the above VO_2 equation becomes:

$$VO_2 = (V_I \times F_IO_2) - (V_E \times F_EO_2)$$

Where:
VO_2 = volume of oxygen consumed per minute
V_I = volume of inspired air per minute
V_E = volume of expired air per minute
F_IO_2 = fraction of inspired oxygen[*]
F_EO_2 = fraction of expired oxygen

[*]F_IO_2 is a constant and equals 0.2094

Computation example: What would be the VO_2 (oxygen consumption) for an aerobic dancer who has a V_I equal to 54.3 L/min, a V_E equal to 54.5 L/min, and a F_EO_2 of 0.1605?

$$VO_2 = (54.3 \text{ L/min} \times 0.2094) - (54.5 \text{ L/min} \times 0.1605)$$

$$VO_2 = (11.37 \text{ L/min}) - (8.74 \text{ L/min})$$
$$= 2.63 \text{ L/min}$$

It should be mentioned that oxygen consumption volumes should be corrected and expressed in STPD (ST = standard temperature, P = standard pressure, and D = Dry) so that results are comparable in different environmental conditions. For example, without correction, oxygen consumption values measured in a high temperature, low-pressure environment would be much larger than values measured in a low-temperature, high-pressure environment. Likewise, humidity can alter oxygen consumption results. Thus, to make VO_2 measures meaningful and comparable across different environmental conditions, an STPD correction factor is required to standardize temperature, pressure, and humidity. A typical STPD correction factor is 0.814 (Appendix C).

Computation example: Correct the above VO_2 measure of the aerobic dancer ($VO_2 - 2.7$ L/min) with the STPD correction factor of 0.814.

$$VO_{2STPD} = 2.7 \text{ L/min} \times 0.814 = 2.19 \text{ L/min}$$

The above discussion was intended to introduce the fundamental principles of VO_2 calculations. Through further study and analysis you can come to learn much more about how exercise scientists calculate VO_2 or VO_{2max}. The important thing to know at this point is that oxygen consumption, whether measured at rest or maximal exercise, is based on the simple equation: $VO_2 = V_IO_2 - V_EO_2$.

The MET

VO_{2max} scores are often expressed in METs. One MET is equivalent to an average resting metabolic rate of 3.5 ml·kg·min^{-1}. Because MET scores are multiples of resting metabolism, a 15.7 MET value indicates that exercise metabolism is 15.7 times higher than at rest. MET scores are computed by dividing VO_2 in ml·kg^{-1}·min^{-1} by 3.5. For average college students, maximum MET values generally range between 11.4 and 17.2 (40 to 60 ml·kg^{-1}·min^{-1}).

SELECTED REFERENCES

Adams, G. M. (1990). *Exercise Physiology Lab Manual*. Dubuque, Iowa: Wm. C. Brown Publishers, 1990, pp: 67–78.

American Heart Association: Guidelines for exercise testing (1986). *Circulation* 75:653A–667A.

Borg, G. A. V. (1970). Perceived exertion as an indicator of somatic stress. *Scandinavian Journal of Rehabilitative Medicine* 2:92–98.

Borg, G. A. V. (1973). Perceived exertion: a note on history and methods. *Medicine and Science in Sports* 5(2):90–93.

Fisher, A. G., and C. R. Jensen (1990). *Scientific Basis of Athletic Conditioning* (3rd edition). Philadelphia: Lea & Febiger, pp: 122–136.

Fox, E. L., R. W. Bowers, and M. L. Foss (1988). *The Physiological Basis of Physical Education and Athletics* (4th edition). Philadelphia: Saunders College Publishing, pp: 61–85.

Heyward, V. H. (1991). *Advanced Fitness Assessment and Exercise Prescription*. Champaign, Illinois: Human Kinetics, pp: 18–40.

Kline, G. M., J. P. Porcari, R. Hintermeister, et al. (1987). Estimation of VO_{2max} from a one-mile track walk, by gender, age, and body weight. *Medicine and Science in Sports and Exercise* 19(3):253–259.

Lamb, D. R. (1984). *Physiology of Exercise: Responses and Adaptations* (2nd edition). New York: Macmillan Publishing Company, pp: 173–190.

McArdle, W. D., F. I. Katch, and V. L. Katch (1991). *Exercise Physiology: Energy, Nutrition, and Human Performance* (3rd edition). Philadelphia: Lea & Febiger, pp: 145–157.

Powers, S. K., and E. T. Howley (1990). *Exercise Physiology: Theory and Application to Fitness and Performance*. Dubuque, Iowa: Wm. C. Brown Publishers, pp: 428–430.

Taylor, H., E. Buskirk, and A. Henschel (1955). Maximal oxygen intake as an objective measure of cardiorespiratory performance. *J. Appl. Physiol* 8:73–80.

Wilmore, J. H., and D. L. Costill, (1988). *Training for Sport and Activity: The Physiological Basis of the Conditioning Process* (3rd edition). Dubuque, Iowa: Wm. C. Brown Publishers, pp: 361–368.

STATION 1

Measurement of VO_{2MAX}

Research Questions

1. Discuss at least three reasons why it is useful to measure VO_{2max}.

2. Describe your test results. Did your subject satisfy the criteria for a VO_{2max} test? What is the fitness rating for your subject based on normative data? (See Chapter 5.)

3. If your subject was advised to exercise at an intensity equal to 70–80% of VO_{2max}, what would be his or her recommended exercise intensity range in $ml \cdot kg^{-1} \cdot min^{-1}$, $kcal \cdot min^{-1}$, and METs? Assume that $1 \, L \, O_2 = 5$ kcals.

4. As a result of an ideal exercise program, VO_{2max} can normally increase no more than 20 percent. If the VO_{2max} of your volunteer were to increase 15%, would this place him or her in a different fitness category? (Show your work.)

5. Could anyone with an ideal exercise program become an elite marathon runner and run 26.2 miles in 2 hrs 20 min? Justify your answer.

Data Collection

Your instructor will supervise the data collection for this lab and may ask for your assistance. Record the data your instructor provides for you on the appropriate data sheet. Outlined below are instructions for a maximal exertion treadmill protocol. (Only slight modifications to these instructions will be necessary if your laboratory is better equipped to perform a maximal cycle ergometer test.)

1. Calibrate the metabolic equipment.
2. Gather preliminary data about your subject (volunteer) prior to testing, such as age, body mass, and height. Record on Chart 12–1. Explain all test procedures to your subject and have him or her sign an informed consent form.
3. Attach appropriate telemetry equipment or ECG electrodes to monitor heart rate.
4. Secure a blood pressure cuff around an arm of the volunteer. Select the arm that will not interfere with treadmill operation. Use athletic tape or duct tape to secure the cuff in place.
5. Measure your subject's resting heart rate and blood pressure (sitting position). Record on Chart 12–1.
6. Have your subject straddle the treadmill belt and hold the front or side rail.

7. Help your subject insert the mouthpiece; tell him or her to make a tight seal around the mouthpiece with his or her lips throughout the entire test.

8. Securely attach nose clips to your subject so as to completely occlude the nostrils.

9. Turn on the treadmill and set the speed at 3.0 mph.
   Instruct your subject to:
   a. hold the treadmill railing when stepping onto the treadmill;
   b. let go of the railing when walking feels comfortable;
   c. look forward at all times (avoid looking down at feet);
   d. stay within arm's reach of the front railing.

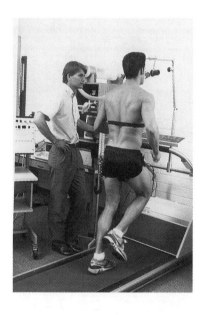

10. Increase the speed of the treadmill. Instruct your subject to provide hand signals (e.g., thumbs up) when the treadmill speed is at a comfortable fast walking pace. (This speed is usually between 3.0 and 4.5 mph.)

11. Allow your subject to walk at this self-selected pace (at a 5% grade) for 3 minutes. During the third minute, measure exercise heart rate and blood pressure. Have your subject look at a duplicate of the RPE scale; have him or her point to the number on the scale that represents his or her subjective appraisal of effort, stress, and fatigue. Record the treadmill speed, heart rate, blood pressure, and RPE for stage 1 on Chart 12–1. Note also any abnormal symptoms.

12. Inform your subject that the treadmill speed will be increased until a comfortable jogging pace is achieved. Have your subject give a thumbs-up sign when the treadmill speed is appropriate. (Most volunteers will likely self-select a speed between 5.0 and 7.5 mph). Less fit subjects can continute to walk if jogging is too strenuous.

13. Have your subject jog at this speed for 3 minutes (level grade). Record the treadmill speed, heart rate, RPE, and blood pressure on Chart 12–1 (stage 2).

14. Continue the test with stages of 1 minute each. Maintain a constant treadmill speed for the remainder of the test. Increase treadmill grade 1.5% every 1 minute until your volunteer reaches volitional fatigue. Within the last minute of each 1-minute stage, record heart rate, blood pressure (when feasible), RPE, and any abnormal symptoms on Chart 12–1.

15. Be prepared to stop the treadmill when your subject reaches volitional fatigue. Tell your subject to raise his or her index finger when he or she feels that he or she has about a minute to go before volitional fatigue.

16. Provide verbal encouragement such as "Work hard," "All the way," "Keep it up." As your subject approaches maximal effort, be aware of safety concerns. Be prepared to stop the treadmill quickly. Make sure your subject stays within arm's reach of the front railing, and, if necessary, place your hand behind the subject to keep him or her near the front end of the treadmill. Do not take a blood pressure reading during the final stages of the test, since this may hinder performance.

17. When your subject indicates that he or she has about a minute to go before volitional fatigue, have a test administrator record the final

treadmill speed and grade. Tell the volunteer to grab the front railing of the treadmill when he or she can run no longer. Record maximal exercise heart rate as your subject completes the test. Decrease the speed and grade of the treadmill to about 2 to 3 mph (level grade) when the subject grabs the front railing.

18. Remove the mouthpiece and noseclips. Allow the volunteer to walk slowly (cool down) for about 6 minutes. Continue to monitor heart rate and blood pressure throughout the 6-minute cool-down period.

A summary of the treadmill protocol is presented in Table 12–4.

19. Compute the subject's VO_{2max} (and correct to STPD) with the test data provided by your instructor. Express your VO_{2max} results in $L \cdot min^{-1}$, $ml \cdot kg^{-1} \cdot min^{-1}$, and METs. Show all work. Determine the fitness classification of your subject, based on age and gender norms outlined in Chapter 5. Record on Chart 12–1.

Table 12–4
Protocol for the Maximal Exercise Test

Stage	Elapsed Time (min)	Treadmill Speed (mph)	Treadmill Grade (%)
1	0–3	Self-selected walking pace	5
2	3–6	Self-selected jogging pace	0
3	6–7	Same speed	1.5
4	7–8	Same speed	3.0
5	8–9	Same speed	4.5
6	9–10	Same speed	6.0
7	10–11	Same speed	7.5
8	11–12	Same speed	9.0
9	12–13	Same speed	10.5
10	13–14	Same speed	12.0
11	14–15	Same speed	13.5
12	15–16	Same speed	15.0
Recovery			
1	0–3	Slow walk (3 mph)	0
2	3–6	Slow walk (3 mph)	0

Computation example: What would be the caloric expenditure (kcal/min) for a VO_2 of 2.5 L O_2/min? Assume that 1 L O_2 = 5 kcals.

Caloric expenditure = 2.5 L O_2/min × 5 kcals/1 L O_2 = 12.5 kcal/min

Note: Cardiologists often conduct stress tests or graded exercise tests (GXTs) to assess their patients' functional capacity. Generally VO_{2max} is not measured during a clinical stress test; rather the primary purpose is to evaluate exercise electrocardiograms and screen for cardiovascular disease. Your instructor may wish to demonstrate standard stress tests (i.e., Balke or Bruce protocol) and discuss how such tests should be administered and evaluated.

Name: _____ Date: _____

Measurement Of VO$_{2max}$
Assignment

Chart 12–1
Measurement of VO$_{2max}$
Data/Computation Sheet

Age: _____ Gender: M/F Weight: _____ lbs; _____ kg

Height: _____ cm Resting heart rate: _____ bpm

Resting blood pressure: _____ (systolic/diastolic)

Predicted maximal heart rate (220–age): _____ bpm

Stage	Time (min)	Speed (mph)	Grade (%)	HR (bpm)	RPE	Blood Pressure/ Symptoms
1	0–3					
2	3–6					
3	6–7					
4	7–8					
5	8–9					
6	9–10					
7	10–11					
8	11–12					
9	12–13					
10	13–14					
11	14–15					
12	15–16					
Recovery						
1	0–3					
2	3–6					

Test results:

Maximum heart rate: _____ bpm

Difference betwen observed and predicted (220–age) HR$_{max}$: _____

Maximum RER: _____ Maximum RPE: _____

Chart 12–1 (continued)

Measurement of VO_{2max}
Data/Computation Sheet

Check the criteria satisfied for VO_{2max} test:

☐   Exercise heart rate no more than 15 bpm below the age-predicted maximum heart rate

☐   Respiratory exchange ratio (RER) ≥ 1.1

☐   Oxygen consumption leveled off despite an increase in work

*VO_{2max} data and computations:

STPD correction factor: _____

V_I: _____ L/min (non-corrected) V_E: _____ L/min

F_IO_2: _____ F_EO_2: _____

(All data considered at maximum exertion)

VO_2 (L O_2/min) = $(V_I \times F_IO_2) - (V_E \times F_EO_2)$

Show your work:

VO_{2max} results:

   VO_{2max} = _____ $ml \cdot kg^{-1} \cdot min^{-1}$ (STPD)

   VO_{2max} = _____ $L \cdot min^{-1}$ (STPD)

   VO_{2max} = _____ METs (STPD)

   Fitness category: _____

*Obtain necessary data from your lab instructor to compute the results. Show all your work.

If available, attach computerized printout of the VO_{2max} test to your lab report.

Research Conclusions

1. Discuss at least three reasons why it is useful to measure VO_{2max}.

2. Describe your test results. Did your subject satisfy the criteria for a VO_{2max} test? What is the fitness rating for your subject based on normative data? (See Chapter 5.)

3. If your subject was advised to exercise at an intensity equal to 70–80% of VO_{2max}, what would be his or her recommended exercise intensity range in $ml \cdot kg^{-1} \cdot min^{-1}$, $kcal \cdot min^{-1}$, and METs? Assume that 1 L $O_2 = 5$ kcals. Show your work.

4. As a result of an ideal exercise program, VO_{2max} can normally increase no more than 20 percent. If the VO_{2max} of your volunteer were to increase 15%, would this place him or her in a different fitness category? (Show work; see norms in Chapter 5.)

5. Could anyone with an ideal exercise program become an elite marathon runner and run 26.2 miles in 2 hrs 20 min? Justify your answer.

. . . .
Lab 12 Summary

Describe several ways the information learned in this lab can be applied to your chosen field of interest and/or your personal life. Be specific and provide practical examples.

13

Pulmonary Function

. . . .
Pre-Laboratory Assignment

1. Describe the difference between lung volume and lung capacity.

2. Draw and label a spirogram of the four lung volumes and four lung capacities.

3. Define vital capacity. What is the predicted vital capacity of a 25-year-old male who is 6 feet 5 inches?

4. What is the %FEV$_{1.0}$ of a person who expired 3872 ml in 1.0 second and has a VC of 4250 ml? Is this score considered normal?

5. ☐ Check the box if you have read each research question for this lab and are familiar with the data collection procedures regarding each research question.

13

Pulmonary Function

The pulmonary system provides an indispensable function for the body at rest and during exercise. Life itself is dependent on the ability of the pulmonary system to deliver oxygen to blood proteins (hemoglobin) and eliminate excess carbon dioxide for maintenance of proper blood pH.

Pulmonary function is generally not considered a limiting factor to aerobic performance at altitudes close to sea level. Thus, the pulmonary system in a normal, healthy individual does not limit one's ability to sustain aerobic exercise for prolonged periods. However, in compromised individuals who have pulmonary disorders (e.g., asthma, emphysema), the pulmonary system can limit functional exercise capacity.

There are primarily two types of pulmonary tests—static and dynamic tests. Static pulmonary tests demonstrate the mechanics of ventilation and are used to quantify the various lung volumes. Dynamic pulmonary tests, on the other hand, are more active in nature and assess the functional ability of the lungs to ventilate air. The dynamic pulmonary tests are commonly used to screen for potential pulmonary disorders such as obstructive lung disease.

Lung Volumes and Capacities
Lung volumes are considered specific entities, whereas lung capacities represent two or more volumes. There are four lung volumes and four lung capacities with which you should be familiar. A spirogram of various lung volumes and capacities is illustrated in Figure 13–1.

Lung Volumes
- Tidal volume (TV): The volume of air inspired (or expired) in a normal breath.

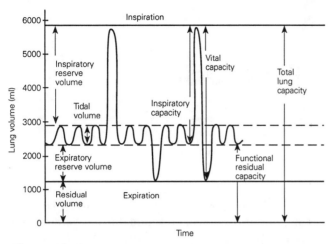

Figure 13–1

- Inspiratory reserve volume (IRV): The maximum volume of air that can be inspired above the tidal volume.
- Expiratory reserve volume (ERV): The maximum volume of air that can be expired below tidal volume.
- Residual volume (RV): The volume of air remaining in the lungs at the end of a maximal expiration.

Lung Capacities
- Vital capacity (VC): The maximum amount of air that can be forcefully expired from the lungs following a maximal inspiration. The sum of tidal volume, inspiratory reserve volume, and expiratory reserve volume; VC = TV + IRV + ERV. When the vital capacity is forced out as fast as possible, it is termed FVC (forced vital capacity).
- Inspiratory capacity (IC): The sum of tidal volume and inspiratory reserve volume; IC = TV + IRV.
- Functional residual capacity (FRC): The amount of air remaining in the lungs after a normal expiration. The sum of expiratory reserve volume and residual volume; FRC = ERV + RV.
- Total lung capacity (TLC): The total amount of air in the lungs after a maximal inspiration. The sum of vital capacity and residual volume; TLC = VC + RV.

Typical lung volumes and capacities are presented in Table 13–1.

Equipment
Pulmonary lung volumes and capacities can be measured with a wet (water-filled) spirometer (Figure 13–2). The mode of operation for the spirometer is a rather simple one. For example, as subjects expire into the respiratory tube of a spirometer, a light-weight plastic or metal bell will rise and move an attached recording pen. The distance the pen moves as recorded on standard chart paper will correspond to the volume of expired air. In like fashion, as subjects inspire from the spirometer, the bell will lower, and a recording of inspiratory volume will be made.

The chart paper of a spirometer is positioned on a rotating drum (kymograph). The kymograph or drum can rotate at a slow (60 mm/min) or fast (1200 mm/min) speed. The horizontal axis of the spirogram represents units of time (mm/min), and the vertical axis represents units of volume (ml). The exact units for the chart paper are typically specified on the paper itself. The recording of various pulmonary volumes and capacities is called a spirogram (Figure 13–1).

To ensure that air does not escape during the measurement process, it is important that subjects keep their lips tightly sealed around the mouthpiece, the nostrils of subjects are completely occluded, and the respiratory tubes and spirometer are airtight. If subjects can continue to breathe via the nose with

Table 13–1
Lung Volumes and Capacities*

Measure	Male (ml)	Female (ml)
Tidal volume (TV)	400–600	350–500
Inspiratory reserve volume (IRV)	3100	1900
Expiratory reserve volume (ERV)	1200	800
Residual volume (RV)	1200	1000
Vital capacity (VC)	4800	3200
Inspiratory capacity (IC)	3600	2400
Functional residual capacity (FRC)	2400	1800
Total lung capacity (TLC)	6000	4200

*Typical lung volumes and capacities for healthy subjects aged 20–30 years in recumbent position.

Source: Comroe (1962).

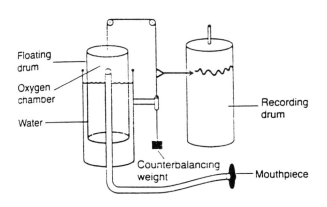

Floating drum
Oxygen chamber
Water
Counterbalancing weight
Recording drum
Mouthpiece

Figure 13–2

noseclips on and mouth closed, the noseclips should be readjusted accordingly.

All equipment (mouthpiece, noseclips, spirometer) used in the measurement process must be properly sanitized. For example, the water in the spirometer should be clean and germ-free. Mouthpieces and noseclips should be scrubbed and placed in a antiseptic solution after use. Always use a clean paper towel when handling mouthpieces prior to use; be sure not to touch mouthpieces with your fingers before they are used by a subject.

Subject Preparation

Subject preparation for pulmonary tests is very minimal. However, it is important that subjects are rested and have sufficient energy to perform the tests (especially the dynamic lung tests) and are free from upper respiratory viral infections (colds) and associated symptoms. Prior to evaluation, subjects should be thoroughly instructed regarding test procedures.

Measurement of TV, IRV, ERV, and VC

The norms provided in Table 13–1 for static pulmonary volumes and capacities are based on subjects who were tested in a recumbent (sitting) position.

Table 13–2
Normal Values for %FEV$_{1.0-3.0}$

Measures	Normal Values
%FEV$_{1.0}$ (FEV$_{1.0}$/FVC)	≥ 83%
%FEV$_{3.0}$ (FEV$_{3.0}$/FVC)	≥ 97%

Source: Consolazio et al. (1963).

Therefore, it is recommended that subjects assume the same position when evaluated.

Because subjects are expected to perform maximal inspirations and expirations during test procedures, it is helpful to provide verbal encouragement for subjects such as "Keep it up," "Push hard," or "You can do it." The timing of such encouragement should occur when subjects reach the top and bottom of vital capacity—when as much air as possible is being drawn in or forced out of the lungs.

Measurement of Forced Vital Capacity (FVC) and Forced Expiratory Volume (FEV$_{1.0-3.0}$)

Individuals with severe lung disease can actually demonstrate normal vital capacity measures if no time limits are placed on the ventilatory maneuver. For this reason, pulmonary specialists use a more dynamic measure of lung function, such as the percentage of vital capacity that can be forcefully expired in one second and/or three seconds. This percentage (%FEV = FEV/FVC) is highly correlated with chronic obstructive pulmonary disease (COPD). Normally, at least 83 percent of vital capacity should be expired in one second and 97 percent of vital capacity in three seconds (Table 13–2). Important factors that can limit the flow rate of expired air are a high flow resistance and poor muscular strength of expiratory muscles. Individuals with severe COPD may exhibit FEV$_{1.0}$ values as low as 20 to 40 percent of FVC.

The measurement of %FEV is performed by taking a maximal inspiration and then, on cue, expiring as fast and as hard as possible into a spirometer. The subject can assume either a standing or sitting position. From the spirogram (spirometer printout) for a %FEV test, both the FEV$_{1.0}$ and/or FEV$_{3.0}$ and FVC can be determined. (Note: Because the spirometer has a known paper speed [1200 mm/min], the volume expired in one second can be ascertained.)

Computation example: What is the %FEV$_{1.0}$ of a person who expires 4305 ml in 1.0 second and has a FVC of 4600 ml? Is this score considered normal?

$$\%FEV_{1.0} = FEV_{1.0}/FVC$$

$$\%FEV_{1.0} = 4305 \text{ ml}/4600 \text{ ml} = 93.5\%, \text{ i.e., normal.}$$

Measurement of RV

The measurement of RV is somewhat more complicated and expensive than the above-mentioned pulmonary tests. The reason for this is that RV cannot be measured directly and requires the use of molecular gases (helium, nitrogen) and expensive equipment (gas analyzers).

The only practical way to measure RV is to utilize proven principles of gas dilution. For example, when a known volume of gas is mixed with an unknown volume of air, the concentration of gas will decrease in proportion to that of the unknown volume. Thus, if 600 ml of helium were added to an unknown (airtight) volume, and the concentration of gas were then measured at 0.10 (10 percent), this would mean that the drop in helium percent (from 100 percent to 10 percent) would be in proportion to that of the unknown volume. Accordingly, the simple calculation of 600 ml divided by 0.10 would equal the unknown volume (600 ml/0.10 = 6,000 ml).

There are several protocols that can be used to measure RV; however, all utilize, in some form, the basic principle of gas dilution discussed above. As a supplement to this lab experience, your instructor may discuss in more detail exactly how RV is measured in your laboratory. A valuable exercise is to study a given RV measurement procedure (and accompanying formula) and be able to conceptualize how each utilizes fundamental principles of gas dilution.

RV is primarily performed in conjunction with hydrostatic weighing to allow for computation of body density and percent body fat. RV can be predicted (see equation and computation example below) with acceptable accuracy; however, even a 100 ml prediction error in RV can lead to large errors in percent fat calculations. Therefore, whenever possible, RV should be measured via gas dilution to improve the accuracy of hydrostatic weighing.

Gas Volume Correction

Lung volumes and capacities should always be corrected and expressed in terms of BTPS (BT = body temperature; P = atmospheric pressure; S = saturated). The reason for this is that a given volume of air in the lungs normally does not equal the same volume of air in a spirometer. Thus, as air is expired from the lungs into a spirometer, the air actually shrinks in size (decreases in volume). Conversely, as air is taken into the lungs it enlarges and increases in volume.

The primary reason for this change in volume between lungs and spirometer is a change in temperature. Normally, room air is about 22°C and body temperature 37°C, and since gas expands as it is heated, this accounts for the volume increase. (Note that when room temperature is above 37°C, this relationship will reverse. Also note that because atmospheric pressure is the same in both lungs and spirometer, no correction is necessary for this variable.) Accordingly, the BTPS correction factor adjusts (increases) the spirometer measures so that actual lung volumes are represented. A typical BTPS correction factor is 1.075 (Appendix C).

Computation example: A spirogram indicates that a female subject has a VC of 3,150 ml. Assuming a BTPS correction factor of 1.075, what would be her actual VC (within the lungs)?

$$VC_{BTPS} = 3{,}150 \text{ ml} \times 1.075 = 3{,}386.2 \text{ ml}$$

Prediction of Lung Volumes and Capacities

Lung volumes and capacities can be predicted from regression equations in the same way that health-related fitness measures are predicted. Important predictor variables in the estimation of lung volumes and capacities are gender, age, and height. Although aerobic training has been shown to alter pulmonary measures, it has not been used to help predict lung volumes and capacities.

Outlined below are prediction equations for both vital capacity and residual volume.

Vital capacity (VC) prediction equation (Baldwin, 1948):

Males:

$$VC_{BTPS} \text{ (ml)} = [27.63 - (0.112 \times age)] \times height;cm$$

Females:

$$VC_{BTPS} \text{ (ml)} = [21.78 - (0.101 \times age)] \times height;cm$$

Computation example: What is the predicted vital capacity of a 23-year-old female who is 5 feet 8 inches?

$$VC_{BTPS} \ (ml) = [21.78 - (0.101 \times 23)] \times 172.7 \ cm$$

$$VC_{BTPS} \ (ml) = 19.45 \times 172.7 = 3360.2 \ ml$$

Residual Volume (RV) prediction equation (Goldman and Becklace, 1959):

Males:

$$RV_{BTPS} \ (L) = 0.017 \ (age)$$
$$+ \ 0.06858 \ (height; inches) - 3.477$$

Females:

$$RV_{BTPS} \ (L) = 0.009 \ (age)$$
$$+ \ 0.08128 \ (height; inches) - 3.90$$

Computation example: What is the predicted residual volume of a 30-year-old male who is 5 feet 11 inches?

$$RV_{BTPS} \ (L) = 0.017 \ (30) + 0.06858 \ (71) - 3.477$$

$$RV_{BTPS} \ (L) = 0.51 + 4.87 - 3.477 = 1.9 \ L$$

SELECTED REFERENCES

Adams, G. M. (1990). *Exercise Physiology Lab Manual*. Dubuque, Iowa: Wm. C. Brown Publishers, pp: 149–165.

Baldwin, E. (1948). *Medicine* 27:243.

Consolazio, C. F., R. E. Johnson, and L. J. Pecora (1963). *Physiological Measurements of Metabolic Functions in Man*. New York: McGraw-Hill, p: 225.

Comroe, J. H., R. E. Farster, and A. B. Dubois (1965). *The Lung: Clinical Physiology and Pulmonary Function Tests* (2nd edition). Chicago: Year Book Medical Publishers, Inc.

DeVries, H. A. (1986). *Physiology of Exercise: For Physical Education and Athletics* (4th edition). Dubuque, Iowa: Wm. C. Brown Publishers.

Fisher, A. G., and C. R. Jensen (1990). *Scientific Basis of Athletic Conditioning* (3rd edition). Philadelphia: Lea & Febiger, pp: 101–108.

Fox, E. L., R. W. Bowers, and M. L. Foss (1988). *Physiological Basis of Physical Education and Athletics* (4th edition). Philadelphia: Saunders College Publishing, pp: 204–214.

Goldman, H. L., and M. R. Becklace (1959). Respiratory function tests: normal values of medium altitude and the prediction of normal results. *Am. Rev. Tuber. Respir. Dis.* 79: 457–469.

Lamb, D. R. (1984). *Physiology of Exercise: Responses and Adaptations* (2nd edition). New York: Macmillan Publishing Company, p: 168.

McArdle, W. D., F. I. Katch, and V. L. Katch (1991). *Exercise Physiology: Energy, Nutrition, and Human Performance* (3rd edition). Philadelphia: Lea & Febiger, pp: 281–284.

Powers, S. K., and E. T. Howley (1990). *Exercise Physiology: Theory and Application to Fitness and Performance*. Dubuque, Iowa: Wm. C. Brown Publishers, pp: 205–216.

Wilmore, J. H., and D. L. Costill (1988). *Training for Sport and Activity: The Physiological Basis of the Conditioning Process* (3rd edition). Dubuque, Iowa: Wm. C. Brown Publishers, pp: 43–46.

STATION 1
. . . .
Pulmonary Function

Research Questions

1. How does the TV, IRV, ERV, and VC of a young, fit college student compare to standard measures in Table 13–1? Describe at least three possible reasons why there may be differences in this comparison.

2. Are predictions of vital capacity (and/or residual volume) for a young, fit college student within $\pm$ 100 ml of actual measures? Provide at least three ways to minimize prediction errors.

3. Are the percent forced expiratory volumes ($\%FEV_{1.0-3.0}$) of a young, fit college student considered normal? Provide at least two reasons why someone might not demonstrate a normal FEV.

Data Collection

Your lab instructor will demonstrate how to perform the various pulmonary tests and may ask for your assistance. Record the test results on the appropriate data sheet.

Name: _____   Date: _____

Pulmonary Function
Assignment

Chart 13–1			
Comparison of Static Lung Measures*			
Gender: Male ☐ Female ☐ Age: _____			
Body Weight: _____ lbs _____ kg Height: _____ inch _____ cm			
Measure	Observed Value (ml)	Standard Value (ml)	Difference (ml)
TV			
IRV			
ERV			
VC			

*All values corrected to BTPS.

Research Conclusions

1. How do the TV, IRV, ERV, and VC of a young, fit college student compare to standard measures in Table 13–1? Describe at least three possible reasons why there may be differences in this comparison.

Chart 13–2			
Observed vs. Predicted Static Lung Measures*			
Gender: Male ☐ Female ☐ Age: _____			
Body Weight: _____ lbs _____ kg Height: _____ inch _____ cm			
Measure	Predicted Value (ml)	Observed Value (ml)	Difference (ml)
VC			
RV			

*All values corrected to BTPS.

2. Are predictions of vital capacity (and/or residual volume) for a young, fit college student within ± 100 ml of actual measures? Provide at least three ways to minimize prediction errors.

Chart 13–3 Dynamic Pulmonary Test Results			

Gender: Male ☐   Female ☐   Age: _____

Body Weight: _____ lbs _____ kg   Height: _____ inch _____ cm

Measure	Observed Score	Criterion for Normal Score	Rating*
% $FEV_{1.0}$			
% $FEV_{3.0}$			

+Data: $FEV_{1.0}$ = _____ ml (BTPS)

$FEV_{3.0}$ = _____ ml (BTPS)

FVC = _____ml (BTPS)

Calculations: (Show work)

*Rating: Specify as normal or abnormal.
+Obtain necessary data from your lab instructor to compute the results. Show all work.

3. Are the percent forced expiratory volumes (% $FEV_{1.0-3.0}$) of a young, fit college student considered normal? Provide at least two reasons why someone might not demonstrate a normal FEV.

Name: _____   Date: _____

. . . .
Lab 13 Summary

Describe several ways the information learned in this lab can be applied to your chosen field of interest and/or your personal life. Be specific and provide practical examples.

Appendix A

Cardiopulmonary Resuscitation (CPR) for Adults and Children

Basic Life Support for an Adult Victim

R   Responsive?

A   Activate the EMS system (usually call 911).

P   Position victim on back.

A   Airway open (use head-tile/chin-lift or jaw thrust).

B   Breathing check (look, listen, and feel for 3–5 seconds).
  • If breathing and spinal injury not suspected, place in recovery position.
  • If not breathing, give 2 slow breaths; watch chest rise.
    – If 2 breaths go in, proceed to step C.
    – If 2 breaths did not go in, retilt head and try 2 more breaths.
    – If second 2 breaths did not go in, give 5 abdominal thrusts; perform tongue-jaw lift followed by a finger sweep; give 2 more breaths. Repeat thrusts, sweep, breaths sequence.

C   Circulation check (at carotid pulse for 5–10 seconds).
  • If there is a pulse but no breathing, give rescue breathing (1 breath every 5–6 seconds).
  • If there is no pulse, give CPR (cycles of 15 chest compressions followed by 2 breaths).

After 1 minute (4 cycles of CPR or 10–12 breaths of rescue breathing), check pulse.
  • If no pulse, give CPR (15:2 cycles), starting with chest compressions.
  • If there is a pulse but no breathing, give rescue breathing.

Basic Life Support for a Child or Infant Victim

E   Establish unresponsive.

S   Send bystander, if available, to activate the EMS system (usually call 911).

P   Position victim on back.

A   Airway open (use head-tile/chin-life or jaw thrust).

B   Breathing check (look, listen, and feel for 3–5 seconds).
  • If breathing and spinal injury not suspected, place in recovery position.
  • If not breathing, give 2 slow breaths; watch chest rise.
    – If 2 breaths go in, proceed to step C.
    – If 2 breaths did not go in, retilt head and try 2 more breaths.
    – If second 2 breaths did not go in, then…

For a child: give 5 abdominal thrusts; perform tongue-jaw lift, and if object is seen perform a finger sweep; give 2 more breaths. Repeat thrusts, mouth check, breaths sequence.

For an infant: give 5 back blows and 5 chest thrusts; perform tongue-jaw lift, and if object is seen perform a finger sweep; give 2 more breaths. Repeat blows, thrusts, mouth check, breaths.

C Circulation check (for 5–10 seconds)
- *For a child:* at carotid pulse; *for an infant:* at brachial pulse.
- If there is a pulse but no breathing, give rescue breathing (1 breath every 3 seconds).
- If there is no pulse, give CPR (cycles of 5 chest compressions followed by 2 breaths).

After 1 minute (10 cycles of CPR or 20 breaths of rescue breathing), check pulse.
- If alone, activate the EMS system.
- If no pulse, give CPR (5:1 cycles), starting with chest compressions.
- If there is a pulse but no breathing, give rescue breathing.

Source: National Safety Council, *CPR Manual*, 1993.

Appendix B

Expression of Data

Today, most scientific publications require that measurements be expressed with metric and SI (Systéme International d'Unités) units. The rationale for this requirement is that metric and SI units provide a universal standard unit of measure and allow easy comparison of quantities.

The units of measure for the metric system relate to one another by powers of 10. Outlined below are typical metric units and their assigned quantities.

nano (n)	one trillionth (10^{-9})
micro (μ)	one millionth (10^{-6})
milli (m)	one thousandth (10^{-3})
centi (c)	one hundredth (10^{-2})
deci (d)	one tenth (10^{-1})
deca(da)	ten (10^{1})
hecto(h)	hundred (10^{2})
kilo(k)	thousand (10^{3})
mega(M)	million (10^{6})
giga(G)	trillion (10^{9})

In the metric system, 1 meter in length is the same as 10 decimeters, 100 centimeters, 1000 millimeters, and so on. One meter is also equivalent to 0.1 decameters, 0.01 hectometers, or 0.001 kilometers. Because it would be awkward to express 100 kilograms as 1000 hectograms, or to refer to a 10 kilometer race as a 0.01 megameter race, the scientific community has established preferred units to express commonly measured parameters. Accordingly, data ought to be expressed in the accepted SI units. In exercise science, a few common SI units include:

distance	kilometer (km)
mass	kilogram (kg)
density	gram per cubic centimeter ($g \cdot cm^{-3}$)
time	second (s)
power	watts (W)
amount of substance	mole (mol)
volume	liter (L)

There are also correct and incorrect ways to express SI units. For example:

1. Body weight should be referred to as body mass (kg), height as stature (m), and skinfold thicknesses as width (mm).
2. SI units should be expressed in singular form and not be pluralized. Thus, although a person weighs more than one kilogram and is taller than one meter, only the singular form is used.
3. SI units should not be followed by a period unless the abbreviation falls at the end of a sentence.
4. SI units should be expressed with an abbreviated symbol, even when values appear within a sentence (e.g., 70 mm, not 70 millimeters).
5. The expression *per* in combined units should be expressed with a negative exponent. For instance, the expression liters per min should be written as $L \cdot min^{-1}$ rather than L/min. The solidus (/), however, can be used in certain instances when it is impractical for a given computer or typewriter to denote the negative exponent expression.
6. SI units should be expressed in a lower-case (noncapitalized) form. An exception to this rule is when the name of the unit is derived from someone's name (e.g., W = watt) or when liters (L) are used to describe a volume. The rationale for the use of a capital L is to prevent confusion with the numeral 1.
7. When the quantity of measurement is smaller than one, it should be expressed as a decimal (with a zero in front of the decimal) rather than a fraction.
8. A space should always be present between the numeral and the symbol.

Examples of correct and incorrect presentation of units are shown below.

	Incorrect Style	Correct Style
90 kilograms	90 kgs	90 kg
85 kilograms	85 K	85 kg
1.82 meters	1.82 ms	1.82 m
10 meters	10 m.	10 m
50 milliliters per kilogram per minute	50 mls/kg/min	50 ml·kg^{-1}·min^{-1}
5 liters	5L	5 L
½ liter	.5 L	0.5 L

In addition, you should also become familiar with normal resting and exercise values of commonly measured physiological parameters. Outlined in Table B–1 are various measures commonly encountered in exercise science. Normal values are listed for both rest and exercise.

SELECTED REFERENCES

Adams, G. M. (1990), *Exercise Physiology Lab Manual*. Dubuque, Iowa: Wm. C. Brown Publishers, p: 234.

Young, D.S. (1987). Implementation of SI units for clinical laboratory data, *Annals of Internal Medicine*, 106(1):114–29.

Table B–1
Normal Values
Expressed with Standard Unit of Measure

Component	Resting Value	Maximal Exercise Value
Heart Rate (bpm)	60–72	190
Systolic blood pressure (mm Hg)	120	200
Diastolic blood pressure (mm Hg)	80	80
Tidal Volume (mL)	500	2,500
V_E (L·min^{-1})	5	120–200
Inspired oxygen (F_IO_2)	0.2094	0.2094
Expired oxygen (F_EO_2)	0.15–0.16	0.145–0.185
VO$_2$ (L·min^{-1})	0.25	4–5
VO$_2$ (ml·kg^{-1}·min^{-1})	3.5	40–80

Appendix C
Gas Volume Correction

Table C–1
STPD Correction Factors

Barometric Pressure (mm Hg)	Room Temperature (°C)					
	Higher Altitude					
	19	20	21	22	23	24
640	.7670	.7632	.7591	.7552	.7511	.7470
642	.7695	.7656	.7616	.7576	.7535	.7494
644	.7719	.7681	.7640	.7601	.7559	.7518
646	.7744	.7705	.7664	.7625	.7583	.7542
648	.7769	.7730	.7689	.7649	.7608	.7566
650	.7793	.7754	.7713	.7674	.7632	.7591
652	.7818	.7779	.7738	.7698	.7656	.7615
654	.7842	.7803	.7762	.7722	.7681	.7639
656	.7867	.7828	.7787	.7747	.7705	.7663
	Lower Altitude					
740	.8900	.8858	.8813	.8770	.8724	.8679
742	.8925	.8882	.8837	.8794	.8748	.8703
744	.8950	.8907	.8862	.8818	.8773	.8727
746	.8974	.8931	.8886	.8843	.8797	.8752
748	.8999	.8956	.8911	.8867	.8821	.8776
750	.9023	.8980	.8935	.8891	.8846	.8800
752	.9048	.9005	.8959	.8916	.8870	.8824
754	.9073	.9029	.8984	.8940	.8894	.8848
756	.9097	.9054	.9008	.8964	.8918	.8873

STPD correction factors can also be computed with the following formula:

$$STPD = [273° + (273° + T_A) \times [(BP - P_{H_2O}) / 760]$$

Where: T_A = Ambient (room) temperataure in °C

P_B = Barometric pressure in mm Hg

P_{H_2O} = Water vapor in mm Hg*

*See Table C–3 for water vapor pressure values

Table C–2
BTPS Correction Factors*

T (°C)	BTPS	T (°C)	BTPS
19	1.107	28	1.057
20	1.102	29	1.051
21	1.096	30	1.045
22	1.091	31	1.039
23	1.085	32	1.032
24	1.080	33	1.026
25	1.075	34	1.020
26	1.068	35	1.014
27	1.063	36	1.007

*The above BTPS correction factors have been computed based on a barometric pressure of 760 mm Hg, the room temperature as listed, and a wet gas (P_{H2O} = 100% relative humidity). Only minimal error is introduced when measurements are conducted at a barometric pressure other than 760 mm Hg. The formula below can also be used to compute BTPS correction factors.

$$BTPS = [(310/(273° + T_A)] \times [(P_B - P_{H_2O_S}) / (P_B - P_{H_2O_B})]$$

Where: T_A = Ambient (room) temperataure in °C

T_B = Body temperature in °C

P_B = Barometric pressure in mm Hg

$P_{H_2O_S}$ = Water vapor in mm Hg* in spirometer

$P_{H_2O_B}$ = Water vapor in mmHg* in lungs (47.1 mm Hg)

*See Table C–3 for water vapor pressure values

Table C–3
Water Vapor Pressure (P_{H2O}; 100% saturated) at Given Temperature

°C	P_{H_2O} mm Hg	°C	P_{H_2O} mm Hg
19	16.5	30	31.8
20	17.5	31	33.7
21	18.7	32	35.7
22	19.8	33	37.7
23	21.1	34	39.9
24	22.4	35	42.2
25	23.8	36	44.6
26	25.2	37	47.1
27	26.7	38	49.7
28	28.4	39	52.4
29	30.0	40	55.3

Appendix D
Sample Computations and Solutions

Metric Conversions

1. What is the kilogram weight of an individual who weighs 132 lbs?

2. What is the centimeter height of an individual who is 4 feet 10 inches? Also, convert this person's height from centimeters to meters.

Muscular Fitness

3. As a test of muscular strength, one male (weighing 80 kg) was able to bench press 120 kg as a 1 RM and 100 kg as a 10 RM. Another male (weighing 70 kg) was able to bench press 90 kg as a 1 RM and 75 kg as a 10 RM. Evaluate and compare the strength of the two men.

4. A college-age female has been strength training as part of a regular exercise regimen in preparation for an upcoming athletic event. She reports to you the following information: Originally her 1 RM and 10 RM leg press was 220 lbs and 180 lbs, respectively. Her current 1 RM and 10 RM leg press is 240 lbs and 210 lbs. She is disappointed that her strength has only improved 20 lbs in the leg press. How can you evaluate her results in a meaningful way?

Heart Rate

5. If a person palpates a 10-second pulse immediately after exercise and measures 27 beats, what is his or her heart rate in beats per minute?

6. If a person palpates her heart rate and it takes 11 seconds for 30 beats to occur, what is her heart rate in beats per minute?

7. If a person palpated a 6-second pulse of 8 beats and continued to palpate a 1-minute pulse of 70 beats, what is the discrepancy between the two methods and why might this occur?

8. What is the estimated maximum heart rate of a 24 year old?

Cardiorespiratory Endurance

9. A 20-year-old female weighing 120 lbs performs the Forestry Step Test and has a post-exercise pulse count of 34 beats/15 seconds. What are her age-adjusted predicted VO_{2max} and fitness rating?

10. A 40-year-old male weighing 180 lbs performs the Forestry Step Test and has a post exercise pulse count of 40 beats per 15 seconds. What are his age adjusted predicted VO_{2max} and fitness rating?

11. A 140-lb 22-year-old-female completes the Astrand Cycle Test with a 15-second pulse count of 36 beats at a work rate of 600 kpm·min^{-1}. What is her predicted VO_{2max} in L·min^{-1} and ml·kg^{-1}·min^{-1}?

12. A 175-lb 20-year-old male performs the Rockport Walking Test in 13 minutes with a heart rate of 130 bpm. He later completes the George-Fisher Jogging Test in a time of 8:15 with a heart rate of 160 bpm. Compare the results of the two tests for this individual.

Body Composition

13. A 5 feet 10 inches tall 35-year-old male weighing 198 lbs visits a health club and in his preliminary screening is measured to have waist and hip circumference measurements of 38 inches and 36 inches, respectively. What do these preliminary measurements suggest?

14. As part of a fitness evaluation, a 30-year-old, 6 foot tall, 220-lb male undergoes several body measurements. His results are as follows: abdominal circumference, 38 inches; wrist circumference, 8 inches; $\sum$3 skinfolds, 60 mm; and $\sum$7 skinfolds, 140 mm. Compute this person's body composition using the Height-squared index, circumference measurements, and the $\sum$3 and $\sum$7 skinfolds.

15. What would the hydrostatic weighing results be for a 19-year-old female subject based on the following data:

Mass in air (M_a) = 63.3 kg; mass in water (M_w) = 2.2 kg; residual volume = 1.4 L; water temperature = 34 °C; assume intestinal gas (VGI) = 0.1 L. Compute percent fat with the Siri formula.

Muscular Fatigue And Ischemia

16. If a person squeezed a hand-grip dynamometer to determine a 1 RM grip strength of 50 kg and then tried to maintain a 100 percent effort contraction for 1 minute, what would be the decrement in strength if immediately following the 1 minute contraction a second 1 RM was only 35 kg?

Muscular Power

17. A 90-kg male ascends a 1.05-meter vertical height of 6 stairs in 0.45 seconds for the Margaria-Kalamen Power Test. What are his power score and rating?

18. A 140-lb female ascends a 1.03 meter vertical height of 6 stairs in 0.66 seconds for the Margaria-Kalamen Power Test. What are her power score and rating?

19. A 100-kg football player performs a series of muscular power tests, two of which are the Wingate Power Test and the Margaria-Kalamen Power Test. Compute the results for both of these tests. Assume that the time elapsed to ascend 1.03 meters of stairs was 0.42 seconds. Also assume that the cycle ergometer work load was set at 7.5 kg and that pedal revolutions for each 5-second interval equaled 10, 9, 7.5, 5.5, 4, and 3.0 revolutions, respectively.

Measurement of Metabolic Rate

20. What is the predicted BMR of a male who has a body weight of 155 lbs and a height of 5 feet, 5 inches, and is 22 years old? Express your answer in kcal/day, kcal/min, LO_2/min, and $ml·kg^{-1}·min^{-1}$.

21. A person is walking on the treadmill at a speed of 3.5 mph and a grade of 5 percent. What would be the predicted oxygen cost for this person?

22. What is the predicted oxygen cost of running on a treadmill at a speed of 6 mph and 0 percent grade?

23. Consider a person who is running on a treadmill during a graded maximal exercise test at a speed and grade equal to 6.5 mph and 10 percent, respectively. What would be the additional oxygen cost for this person assuming the grade was increased to 15 percent?

24. You are administrating a graded exercise test for an athlete whom you have tested previously. You know that her VO_{2max} is approximately 45 $ml·kg^{-1}·min^{-1}$. She is presently running on the treadmill at a speed of 5 mph and grade of 5 percent. How close is she to her maximal work rate?

25. A male subject's VO_{2max} was measured to be 55 $ml·kg^{-1}·min^{-1}$. From previous testing, he knows that he can maintain a pace of 75 percent of his VO_{2max} for at least 2 hours. If the person were to train on level ground, how fast should he be running? Express your answer in mph and $min·mile^{-1}$.

26. A person's VO_{2max} was measured to be 60 $ml·kg^{-1}·min^{-1}$. An important goal for this individual is to run a marathon (26.2 miles) in under 3 hours in order to qualify for the Boston Marathon. Assume he can maintain a pace for 3 hours that elicits an average VO_2 of 45 $ml·kg^{-1}·min^{-1}$. Also assume the marathon is on level ground. Can this person achieve his goal and complete the race in less than 3 hours?

27. A 143-lb female is pedaling on a stationary Monarch bicycle at a rate of 50 rpm and at a work load of 2 kg. What would be her estimated oxygen cost for this exercise? (The Monarch bicycle flywheel is 6 $m·rev^{-1}$.)

28. Consider a 154-lb female who, as part of a weight reduction program, expends 300 kcal per exercise session, 4 days per week. She uses a Monarch stationary bicycle for exercise. She feels comfortable pedaling at a rate of 70 rpm at a work load of 2 kg. For her, this exercise intensity elicits an RER of 0.84 (kcal to oxygen equivalent of 4.85 $kcal·L^{-1}$). How long must she exercise in order to expend the 300 kcal?

Electrocardiograms

29. An ECG tracing is measured to have 15 mm between consecutive R waves. What is the heart rate (bpm)?

30. An ECG tracing is measured to have 8.5 cardiac cycles in 3 seconds. What is the heart rate (bpm)?

31. A 20-year-old completes a maximal graded exercise test. His ECG at maximal exercise is measured to

have 8 mm between R waves. How well does the age-predicted maximal heart rate (220–age) estimate his observed maximal heart rate?

32. An ECG tracing of a young female reveals a sinus arrhythmia, which means that the heart beats normally but at varying time intervals. Assume that the distance between R waves varies between 18–22 mm at rest. Assume also that additional ECG tracings reveal that 7.75 cardiac cycles occurred in 6 seconds and that a 1-minute ECG tracing displayed 80 beats. Can the distance between two consecutive R waves consistently and accurately determine heart rate for this person? Does the 6 second tracing work well enough to use?

Measurement Of VO$_{2max}$

33. What would be the VO$_2$ (L/min) of a walker who has a V$_I$ equal to 38.5 L/min, a V$_E$ equal to 37.3 L/min, and an F$_E$O$_2$ of 0.1695? Assume a STPD correction factor of 0.7509.

34. What would be the maximum MET score of a male athlete who has a VO$_{2max}$ of 58.7 ml·kg^{-1}·min^{-1}? Show your work.

35. If a person's VO$_{2max}$ was measured to be 55 ml·kg^{-1}·min^{-1}, what would be his or her absolute oxygen consumption? Assume a body mass of 75 kg.

36. During a stationary bicycle ride, a person is consuming oxygen at average rate of 2.5 L·min^{-1}. Assuming an RER value of 0.88 and a kcal to oxygen equivalent of 4.90 kcal·L^{-1}, approximately how many kcalories would be expended in a 60-minute exercise session? Assume a constant exercise intensity.

37. A person's VO$_{2max}$ is measured to be 60 ml·kg^{-1}·min^{-1}. This same person typically trains for prolonged periods of time at a pace that elicits a VO$_2$ of 45 ml·kg^{-1}·min^{-1}. Based on this data, determine this person's relative exercise intensity.

Pulmonary Function

38. A spirogram indicates that a male subject has a VC of 4,800 ml. Assuming a BTPS correction factor of 1.11, what would be his actual VC (within the lungs)?

39. During a fitness evaluation, a female subject had her lung volumes and capacities determined. As-

sume her inspiratory reserve volume equaled 2,000 ml, her tidal volume equaled 450 ml, her expiratory reserve volume equaled 1,000 ml, and her residual volume equaled 900 ml. What would be her total lung capacity?

40. A male subject's vital capacity was measured to be 5.6 liters. During a pulmonary function test, he forcefully expired 4,480 ml in 1 second and 5,490 ml in 3 seconds. What are his forced expiratory volumes for 1 s and 3 s expressed as a percentage of vital capacity?

41. A 25-year-old, 6 foot-tall, 190-lb male, has a measured vital capacity of 5 liters. How does his predicted vital capacity compare to his observed vital capacity?

42. A 24-year-old, 5 foot 6 inch female had her residual volume measured at 1,200 ml. Does the prediction equation above provide an estimation that appears suitable for use during a subsequent hydrostatic weighing test?

SOLUTIONS FOR SAMPLE COMPUTATIONS

Metric Conversions

1. What is the kilogram weight of an individual who weighs 132 lb?

$$132 \text{ lbs} \times \frac{0.4536 \text{ kg}}{1 \text{ lb}} = 59.87 \text{ kg}$$

(Notice that the pounds cancel out.)

2. What is the centimeter height of an individual who is 4 feet 10 inches?

$$4 \text{ feet} = (4 \text{ ft} \times 12 \text{ inch/ft} = 48 \text{ inch})$$
$$+ 10 \text{ inches} = 58 \text{ inches}$$

$$58 \text{ in} \times \frac{2.54 \text{ cm}}{1 \text{ in}} = 147.32 \text{ cm}$$

Convert this person's height from centimeters to meters.

$$147.32 \text{ cm} \times \frac{1 \text{ m}}{100 \text{ cm}} = 1.47 \text{ m}$$

Muscular Fitness

3. In absolute terms, the 80-kg male is the stronger and has the greater endurance, since his 1 RM

and 10 RM are the greater. In relation to their individual body weights, the heavier person has the greater strength per kg of body weight (strength-to-weight ratio of 1.5 compared to 1.28 for the lighter man). In absolute terms, the heavier male also has the greater muscular endurance (10 RM = 100 kg), but both men have equal 10 RMs when the weight is expressed as a percentage of their 1 RM (83%).

4. It is true that this woman's absolute leg strength has increased only 20 lbs (9% improvement) as measured by the leg press. In terms of muscular endurance, though, her 10 RM has increased from 180 lbs to 210 lbs, which is a 16% improvement. In addition, her current 10 RM is 87.5% of her current 1 RM, whereas her starting 10 RM was 81.8% of her original 1 RM. Also, her original 10 RM is 75% of her current 1 RM. Thus, even though she may be disappointed with her muscular strength improvements, she has shown greater improvements in muscular endurance, which may be more advantageous for her depending on her training goals.

Heart Rate

5. If 30 beats are palpated in 10 seconds, then the heart rate is:

$$\frac{27 \text{ beats}}{10 \text{ sec}} \times \frac{60 \text{ seconds}}{1 \text{ min}} = 162 \text{ beats/min}$$

6. If 30 heart beats are palpated in 11 seconds, then the heart rate is:

$$\frac{30 \text{ beats}}{11 \text{ sec}} \times \frac{60 \text{ seconds}}{1 \text{ min}} = 163.6 \text{ beats/min}$$

7. If 8 beats are palpated in 6 seconds and then 73 beats are palpated for 1-minute, then:

$$\frac{8 \text{ beats}}{6 \text{ sec}} \times \frac{60 \text{ seconds}}{1 \text{ min}} = 80 \text{ beats/min}$$

80 bpm is 10 bpm greater than the heart rate counted for 1 minute. The error may result from counting an extra beat with the 6-second timed heart rate method.

8. The predicted maximum heart rate (HR_{max}) for a 24-year-old person would be 196 bpm since estimated HR_{max} equals 220 minus age.

Cardiorespiratory Endurance

9. The 20-year-old, 120-lb female performed the Forestry Step Test with a 15-second post-exercise pulse count of 34 beats. Based on Table 5–3, this corresponds to a non-adjusted VO_{2max} of 40 ml·kg^{-1}·min^{-1}. Since the age correction factor for a 20-year-old is 1.02, her predicted age-adjusted VO_{2max} would be:

$$40 \text{ ml·kg}^{-1}\text{·min}^{-1} \times 1.02 = 40.8 \text{ ml·kg}^{-1}\text{·min}^{-1}$$
$$(\text{normative rating} = \text{Good})$$

10. The 40-year-old, 180-lb male, performed the Forestry Step Test with a 15-second post-exercise pulse count of 40 beats. Based on Table 5–2, this corresponds to a non-adjusted VO_{2max} of 37 ml·kg^{-1}·min^{-1}. Since the age-correction factor for a 40-year-old is 0.93, his predicted age-adjusted VO_{2max} is:

$$37 \text{ ml·kg}^{-1}\text{·min}^{-1} \times 0.93 = 34.41 \text{ ml·kg}^{-1}\text{·min}^{-1}$$
$$(\text{normative rating} = \text{Average})$$

11. The 22-year-old, 140-lb (63.6 kg) female terminates the Astrand Cycle Test at a work rate of 600 kgm·min^{-1} with a 15-second pulse count of 36 beats (144 bpm). Using the Astrand nomogram, draw a line from the ending work load to the appropriate female heart rate value. The line drawn should intersect the estimated VO_{2max} line at 2.7 L·min^{-1}. Since the age correction factor for her is 1.02, her age-adjusted estimated VO_{2max} is:

$$2.7 \text{ L·min}^{-1} \times 1.02 = 2.75 \text{ L·min}^{-1}$$

$$(2.75 \text{ L·min}^{-1} \times \frac{1000 \text{ ml}}{\text{liter}}) \div 63.6 \text{ kg}$$
$$= 43.2 \text{ ml·kg}^{-1}\text{·min}^{-1}$$

12. The 175-lb (79.5 kg) male completed the Rockport Walking Test in 13 minutes (13.0 min) with an ending heart rate of 130 bpm and the George-Fisher Jogging Test in 8:15 minutes (8.25 min) with an ending heart rate of 160 bpm. These data equate to predicted VO_{2max} scores of:

Rockport Walking Test

$$132.6 - (0.17 \times 79.5 \text{ kg}) - (0.39 \times 20 \text{ yrs}) + (6.31)$$
$$- (3.27 \times 13 \text{ min}) - (0.156 \times 130 \text{ bpm})$$
$$= 54.8 \text{ ml·kg}^{-1}\text{·min}^{-1}$$

George-Fisher Jogging Test

$$100.5 + (8.344) - (0.1636 \times 79.5 \text{ kg})$$
$$- (1.438 \times 8.25 \text{ min}) - (0.1928 \times 160 \text{ bpm})$$
$$= 53.12 \text{ ml·kg}^{-1}\text{·min}^{-1}$$

Body Composition

13. The 35-year-old male who is 5 feet 10 inches tall and weighs 198 lbs has waist and hip measurements of 38 and 36 inches, respectively. Based on this data you can calculate his BMI and his waist-to-hip ratio as follows:

BMI:

$$70 \text{ in} \times 2.54 \text{ cm/in} = 177.8 \text{ cm} = 1.77 \text{ m}$$
$$198 \text{ lbs} \times 1 \text{ kg}/2.2 \text{ lb} = 90 \text{ kg}$$

$$90 \text{ kg} \div 1.77^2 \text{ m} = 90 \text{ kg} \div 3.1329 \text{ m}^2$$
$$= 28.72 \text{ kg/m}^2$$

Waist-to-Hip Ratio:

$$38 \text{ in} \div 36 \text{ in} = 1.05$$

This person's BMI score indicates that he is moderately obese (Table 6–2): however, if this is not visually obvious, a body composition evaluation may be justified. The high waist-to-hip ratio classifies this person at a high risk (Table 6–3) for cardiovascular disease. The high waist-to-hip ratio also suggests that his BMI is reasonable.

14. The 6-foot tall (182.8 cm; 18.2 dm), 220-lb (100 kg) male has an abdominal circumference of 38 inches (96.52 cm), a wrist circumference of 8 inches (20.32 cm), and $\sum 3$ and $\sum 7$ skinfold measurements of 60 mm and 140 mm, respectively. Accordingly, his body composition results are as follows:

Height Squared Index:

$$\text{LBM (kg)} = 0.204 \times \text{Height (dm)}^2$$

$$\text{LBM} = 0.204 \times 18.2^2 = 67.57 \text{ kg}$$

$$\text{Percent Body Fat} = \frac{\text{Body Weight (kg)} - \text{LBM (kg)}}{\text{Body Weight (kg)}} \times 100$$

$$(100 - 67.57)/100 \times 100 = 32.4\% \text{ body fat}$$

Circumferences:

$$\text{LBW (kg)} = 41.955 + (1.03876 \text{ body} \times \text{weight (kg)})$$
$$- (0.82816 \times (\text{abdominal-wrist}))$$

$$41.955 + (1.03876 \times 100) - (0.82816 \times (96.52 - 20.32)) = 82.7 \text{ kg}$$

$$\text{Percent Body Fat} = \frac{\text{Body Weight (kg)} - \text{LBM (kg)}}{\text{Body Weight (kg)}} \times 100$$

$$(100 - 82.7)/100 \times 100 = 17.3\% \text{ body fat}$$

$\sum 3$ and $\sum 7$ Skinfolds:

$$\text{Db} \sum 3 = 1.10938 - 0.0008267 (\textstyle\sum 3) + 0.0000016$$
$$(\textstyle\sum 3)^2 - 0.0002574 \text{ (age)}$$

$$1.10938 - 0.0008267 (60) + 0.0000016 (3600)$$
$$- 0.0002574 (30) = 1.0578$$

$$\text{Percent Body Fat} = 4.95/\text{Db} - 4.50 \times 100$$
$$4.95/1.0578 - 4.50 \times 100 =$$
$$17.95\%$$

$$\text{Db} \sum 7 = 1.1120 - 0.00043499 (\textstyle\sum 7) + 0.00000055$$
$$(\textstyle\sum 7)^2 - 0.00028826 \text{ (age)}$$

$$1.1120 - 0.00043499 (140) + 0.00000055 (19600)$$
$$- 0.00028826 (30)$$
$$= 1.0532$$

$$\text{Percent Body Fat} = 4.95/\text{Db} - 4.5 \times 100$$
$$4.95/1.0532 - 4.5 \times 100$$
$$19.98\%$$

15. The percent fat for a 19-year-old female subject using hydrostatic weighing would be:

$$\text{Water density (D}_w) = 0.994403 \text{ (Table 6–4)}$$

$$\text{Total Body Volume (TBV)} = \frac{(\text{Ma} - \text{Mw})}{\text{D}_W} - (\text{RV} + \text{VGI})$$

$$\text{TBV} = \frac{63.3 - 2.2}{0.994403} - (1.4 + 0.1) = 59.94 \text{ L}$$

$$\text{Body density (Db)} = \text{M}_a \div \text{TBV}$$

$$\text{Db} = 63.3 \text{ kg} \div 59.94 \text{ L} = 1.056$$

$$\text{Percent body fat (Siri)} = (4.95/\text{Db}) - 4.50 \times 100$$

$$\%\text{BF} = (4.95/1.056) - 4.50 \times 100 = 18.76\%$$

Muscular Fatigue and Ischemia

16. If a 1 RM hand-grip strength of 50 kg decreased to 35 kg following one minute of sustained con-

traction, the decrement in strength would be 30%.

$$(50 - 35)/50 = 0.30 \text{ or } 30\%$$

Muscular Power

17. The 90-kg male ascended the 1.05 m vertical height of 6 stairs in 0.45 seconds for the Margaria Kalamen Test. His power score and rating are:

$$\text{Power}: \frac{f \times d}{t} = \frac{90 \text{ kg} \times 1.05\text{m}}{0.45\text{s}} = 210 \text{ kgm} \cdot \text{s}^{-1}$$

(normative rating = Good)

18. The 140-lb (63.6 kg) female ascended the 1.03 m vertical height of 6 stairs in 0.66 seconds for the Margaria Kalamen Test. Her power score and rating are:

$$\text{Power}: \frac{f \times d}{t} = \frac{63.6 \text{ kg} \times 1.03 \text{ m}}{0.66\text{s}} = 99.25 \text{ kgm} \cdot \text{s}^{-1}$$

(normative rating = Fair)

19. The 100-kg football player performed the 1.03 m Margaria Kalamen Test in 0.42 seconds. His power score for this test is:

$$\text{Power}: \frac{f \times d}{t} = \frac{100 \text{ kg} \times 1.03 \text{ m}}{0.42 \text{ s}} = 245.2 \text{ kgm} \cdot \text{s}^{-1}$$

(normative rating = Excellent)

For the Wingate Power Test, each 5-second interval equaled 10, 9, 7.5, 5.5, 4, and 3.0 revolutions, respectively.

Cycle ergometer resistance:

$$100 \text{ kg} \times 0.075 = 7.5 \text{ kg}$$

Absolute peak 5-second power (APP):

APP (watts) = load (kg) × peak revolutions × 11.765

$$\text{APP} = 7.5 \text{ kg} \times 10 \text{ rev} \times 11.765 = 882.4 \text{ watts}$$

Relative peak 5-second power (RPP):

$$\text{RPP (watts/kg)} = \text{APP/kg body wt}$$

$$\text{RPP} = 882.4 \text{ watts/100 kg} = 8.82 \text{ watts/kg}$$

Absolute mean 30-second power (AMP):

AMP (watts) = load (kg) × average revolutions × 11.765

Average revolutions per 5-second interval =

$$10 + 9 + 7.5 + 5.5 + 4 + 3.0$$
$$= 39 \text{ revolutions}$$

39 rev/6 intervals of time = 6.5 rev

$$\text{AMP} = 7.5 \text{ kg} \times 6.5 \text{ rev} \times 11.765 = 573.5 \text{ watts}$$

Relative mean 30-second power (RMP):

$$\text{RMP (watts/kg)} = \text{AMP/kg}$$

$$\text{RMP} = 573.5 \text{ watts/100 kg} = 5.74 \text{ watts/kg}$$

Fatigue index (FI):

$$\text{FI} = \frac{\text{Highest peak 5-second power} - \text{lowest peak 5-second power}}{\text{Highest peak 5-second power}}$$

$$\text{FI} = \frac{882.4 \text{ watts} - 264.7 \text{ watts}}{882.4 \text{ watts}} = 0.70 \text{ or } 70\%$$

$$\text{Lowest APP} = 7.5 \text{ kg} \times 3.0 \text{ rev} \times 11.765$$
$$= 264.7 \text{ watts}$$

The athlete's peak power during the first 5 seconds (APP) of the test was 882.4 watts, which is considered a high power output. The relative peak 5-second power (RPP) was 8.82. The absolute mean 30-second power (AMP) was 573.5 watts, which is about at the fifty-fifth percentile (Table 9–3). The relative mean 30-second power (RMP) was 5.73, which is below the tenth percentile (Table 9–3). The athlete's fatigue index was 70%, which is indicative of low endurance. Accordingly, this person has high explosive power, but poor endurance. An educated guess would be that this person has a high percentage of fast-twitch muscle fibers in his quadriceps.

Measurement of Metabolic Rate

20. The predicted BMR for this person would be:

BMR (kcal/day) = 66.47 + (13.75 × body mass;kg)
+ (5.0 × height;cm) − (6.76 × age;yr)

BMR (kcal/day) = 66.47 + (13.75 × 70.45 kg)
+ (5.0 × 165.1 cm) − (6.76 × 22)

BMR (kcal/day) = (66.47 + 968.68 + 825.5) − 148.7
= 1711.94 kcal/day

$$\text{BMR (kcal/min)} = 1711.94 \text{ kcal/day} \times 1 \text{ day/24 hrs} \times 1 \text{ hr/60 min} = 1.188 \text{ kcal/min}$$

$$\text{BMR (L O}_2\text{/min)} = 1.188 \text{ kcal/min} \times 1 \text{ L O}_2\text{/5 kcals} = 0.2376 \text{ L O}_2\text{/min}$$

$$\text{BMR (ml} \cdot \text{kg}^{-1} \cdot \text{min}^{-1})$$
$$= \frac{0.2376 \text{ L O}_2\text{/min} \times 1000 \text{ ml/L O}_2}{70.45 \text{ kg}}$$
$$= 3.37 \text{ ml} \cdot \text{kg}^{-1} \cdot \text{min}^{-1}$$

21. The oxygen cost of walking on the treadmill at 3.5 mph at a 5% grade can be determined using the ACSM walking equation. Be sure to first convert speed in mph to m·min^{-1}.

$$\text{VO}_2 \text{ ml} \cdot \text{kg}^{-1} \cdot \text{min}^{-1} = (\text{walking speed} \times 0.1) + (\text{grade} \times \text{speed} \times 1.8) + (3.5)$$

Speed: treadmill speed expressed as m·min^{-1}
(1 mph = 26.8 m·min^{-1})

Grade: expressed as a decimal (e.g., 10% grade = 0.10)

$$\text{VO}_2 = (93.8 \text{ m·min}^{-1} \times 0.1) + (.05 \times 93.8 \times 1.8) + (3.5) = 21.3 \text{ ml·kg}^{-1}\text{·min}^{-1}$$

22. The oxygen cost of running on the treadmill at 6 mph at a 0% grade can be determined using the ACSM walking equation. Be sure to first convert speed in mph to m·min^{-1}.

$$\text{VO}_2 \text{ ml} \cdot \text{kg}^{-1} \cdot \text{min}^{-1} = (\text{running speed} \times 0.2) + (\text{grade} \times \text{speed} \times 1.8 \times 0.5) + (3.5)$$

Speed: treadmill speed expressed as m·min^{-1}
(1 mph = 26.8 m·min^{-1})

Grade: expressed as a decimal
(e.g., 10% grade = 0.10)

$$\text{VO}_2 = (160.8 \text{ m·min}^{-1} \times 0.2) + (0 \times 160.8 \times 1.8 \times 0.5) + (3.5) = 35.6 \text{ ml·kg}^{-1}\text{·min}^{-1}$$

23. The oxygen cost of running on the treadmill at a speed of 6.5 mph at a 10% grade is:

$$\text{VO}_2 \text{ ml} \cdot \text{kg}^{-1} \cdot \text{min}^{-1} = (\text{running speed}) \times (0.2) + (\text{grade} \times \text{speed} \times 1.8 \times 0.5) + (3.5)$$

Speed: treadmill speed expressed as m·min^{-1}
(1 mph = 26.8 m·min^{-1})

Grade: expressed as a decimal
(e.g., 10% grade = 0.10)

$$\text{VO}_2 = (174.2 \text{ m·min}^{-1} \times 0.2) + (0.1 \times 174.2 \times 1.8 \times 0.5) + (3.5) = 54 \text{ ml·kg}^{-1}\text{·min}^{-1}$$

The oxygen cost of running at the same speed but at 15% grade is:

$$(174.2 \text{ m·min}^{-1} \times 0.2) + (0.15 \times 174.2 \times 1.8 \times 0.5) + (3.5) = 61.8 \text{ ml·kg}^{-1}\text{·min}^{-1}$$

Therefore, the additional oxygen cost for the 5% increase in grade would equal 7.8 ml·kg^{-1}·min^{-1}.

24. The athlete's current oxygen cost of running on the treadmill at 5 mph, 5% grade is calculated with the ACSM equations. Be sure to first convert speed to m·min^{-1}.

$$\text{VO}_2 \text{ ml} \cdot \text{kg}^{-1} \cdot \text{min}^{-1} = (\text{running speed} \times 0.2) + (\text{grade} \times \text{speed} \times 1.8 \times 0.5) + (3.5)$$

Speed: treadmill speed expressed as m·min^{-1}
(1 mph = 26.8 m·min^{-1})

Grade: expressed as a decimal
(e.g., 10% grade = 0.10)

$$\text{VO}_2 = (134 \text{ m·min}^{-1} \times 0.2) + (0.05 \times 134 \times 1.8 \times 0.5) + (3.5) = 36.3 \text{ ml·kg}^{-1}\text{·min}^{-1}$$

If her VO$_{2max}$ is 45 ml·kg^{-1}·min^{-1}, then she is currently working at 80% of her maximal capacity and an increase in speed of 1.3 mph would elicit her VO$_{2max}$.

25. Using the ACSM running equation, you can rearrange the formula and solve for speed. Since you know his VO$_{2max}$ is 55 ml·kg^{-1}·min^{-1} and that he is going to run a pace that elicits 75% of his VO$_{2max}$, then he will be running at an oxygen cost of:

$$55 \text{ ml·kg}^{-1}\text{·min}^{-1} \times 75\% = 41.25 \text{ ml·kg}^{-1}\text{·min}^{-1}$$

Assuming he trains on level ground, solve for speed:

$$41.25 \text{ ml·kg}^{-1}\text{·min}^{-1} = (\text{speed} \times 0.2) + (0 \times \text{speed} \times 1.8 \times 0.5) + 3.5$$

$$41.25 \text{ ml·kg}^{-1}\text{·min}^{-1} = (\text{speed} \times 0.2) + 3.5$$

$$37.75 \text{ ml·kg}^{-1}\text{·min}^{-1} = (\text{speed} \times 0.2)$$

$$188.75 \text{ m·min}^{-2} = \text{speed}$$

Since the speed is expressed in m·min^{-1}, you should now convert this number to mph. To do this, divide by 26.8; the resulting speed equals approximately 7 mph. Since it is difficult to conceptualize what 7 mph really means, running speed or pace can be expressed in terms of how many minutes it takes to run one mile (min·mile^{-1}). If this person were to run at 7 mph, what would his 1-mile pace be?

You should be able to see that 7 mph is the same as 7 miles per 60 minutes, which is the same as 0.1167 miles per minute (7 miles ÷ 60 minutes). The inverse of 0.1167 miles·min^{-1} is 8.57 min·mile^{-1}. Accordingly, he should run at a pace of about 8.5 min·mile^{-1} in order to run at 75% of his VO$_{2max}$.

26. This is a very practical application of the ACSM equations. As in problem 25, use the ACSM equation and solve for speed. Once speed (m·mile^{-1}) is computed, determination of the time it would take to run the 26.2 miles is a simple matter of multiplication or division. Of course, in a real life situation, we must also consider other factors, such as training, nutrition, hydration, temperature, humidity, terrain, and the like. However, this computation provides a good approximation.

Solve for speed first:

$$45 \text{ ml·kg}^{-1}\text{·min}^{-1} = (\text{speed} \times 0.2) + (0 \times \text{speed} \times 1.8 \times 0.5) + 3.5$$

$$45 \text{ ml·kg}^{-1}\text{·min}^{-1} = (\text{speed} \times 0.2) + 3.5$$

$$41.5 \text{ ml·kg}^{-1}\text{·min}^{-1} = (\text{speed} \times 0.2)$$

$$207.5 \text{ m·min}^{-2} = \text{speed}$$

Convert the speed 207.5 m·min^{-1} to 7.74 mph by dividing by 26.8. Now determination of whether or not the person can complete the 26.2-mile marathon can be done in one of two ways. A first alternative is to convert the speed to a mile·min^{-1} pace (0.129). Then, since there are 180 minutes in 3 hours, multiply by 180:

$$0.129 \text{ mile·min}^{-1} \times 180 \text{ min} = 23.2 \text{ miles}$$

Thus, at a speed of 7.74 mph, the person would only be able to run 23.2 miles in the 3-hour time period and would not be able to complete the marathon in a qualifying time.

A second alternative is to use the running speed to determine how long it would actually take to finish the race. Accordingly, at a pace of 0.129 mile·min^{-1}, how long would it take to run 26.2 miles?

$$26.2 \text{ miles} \div 0.129 \text{ mile·min}^{-1} = 203 \text{ minutes}$$
$$= 3.38 \text{ hours} = 3 \text{ hr } 23 \text{ min}$$

27. The oxygen cost of pedaling on a cycle ergometer can be determined with the ACSM equations. For cycle ergometer equations, pedal speed (rpm) and resistance must be known. The circumference of the flywheel is constant and for a Monarch cycle ergometer is 6 meters per revolution.

$$VO_2 \text{ ml·min}^{-1} = (\text{kg} \times \text{m/rev} \times \text{rev/min}) \times (2)$$
$$+ (3.5 \times \text{body weight})$$

$$VO_2 = (2 \text{ kg} \times 6 \text{ m·rev}^{-1} \times 50 \text{ rev·min}^{-1}) \times (2)$$
$$+ (3.5 \times 65 \text{ kg}) = 1427 \text{ ml·min}^{-1}$$

28. To calculate how long it will take this female to expend approximately 300 kcal, you must first know her rate of oxygen consumption and the rate of calorie expenditure. To compute the former value, you can use the ACSM equation, and the latter value is provided for you.

$$(2 \text{ kg} \times 6 \text{ m·rev}^{-1} \times 70 \text{ rev·min}^{-1}) \times (2)$$
$$+ (3.5 \times 70 \text{ kg}) = 1925 \text{ ml·min}^{-1} = 1.92 \text{ L·min}^{-1}$$

If the kcal to oxygen equivalent is 4.85 kcal·L^{-1}, then the caloric expenditure per minute is:

$$1.92 \text{ L·min}^{-1} \times 4.85 \text{ kcal·L}^{-1} = 9.3 \text{ kcal·min}^{-1}$$

If the objective is to expend 300 kcal, then it will take

$$300 \text{ kcal} \div 9.3 \text{ kcal·min}^{-1} = 32.25 \text{ min}$$

Electrocardiograms

29. Each 1-mm interval on the horizontal axis of the ECG paper represents 0.04 seconds at a paper speed of 25 mm·s^{-1} (1 s ÷ 25 mm). This would also mean there are 1,500 mm·min^{-1} (60 s × 25 mm· s^{-1}) at this same paper speed. Knowing this information, one can count the distance between consecutive cardiac cycles to determine heart rates from ECG tracings. Accordingly, if there were 15 mm between two consecutive cardiac cycles, then:

$$1500 \text{ mm·min}^{-1} \div 15 \text{ mm·beat}^{-1}$$
$$= 100 \text{ beats·min}^{-1} \text{ (bpm)}$$

30. Another way to determine heart rates from ECG tracings is to count the number of cardiac cycles in an allotted period of time, such as 3 seconds, and then multiply by the correct factor to get minute-heart rates. For example, when measuring the number of cardiac cycles in 3 seconds, you should multiply by 20 (3 s × 20 = 60 s = 1 min). Thus, if there were 8.5 cardiac cycles in 3 seconds, the minute heart rate would be:

$$8.5 \text{ beats} \times 20 = 170 \text{ bpm}$$

31. Determine the heart rate at maximal exercise by dividing 1,500 mm·min⁻¹ by 8 mm·beat⁻¹. Compare this heart rate to his age predicted maximal heart rate (220–age).

Observed maximal HR: $1{,}500 \text{ mm·min}^{-1}$
$\div 8 \text{ mm·beat}^{-1} = 187.5 \text{ bpm}$

Age predicted maximal HR: 220 – 20 = 200 bpm

This person's actual maximal HR is about 95% of his age-predicted HR. He should, therefore, use his observed maximal HR for determining his target heart rate training zone.

32. Using the distance between cardiac cycles is a good method for determining heart rate from ECG tracings only when the cardiac rhythm is normal. In cases in which it is not normal, the number of cycles that occur in 3, 6, or 10 seconds should be used. In this problem, measurement error will result if the interval between two consecutive cardiac cycles is used to determine heart rate from the ECG tracing. An interval of 18–22 mm between cardiac cycles computes to a resting heart rate of between 68 bpm and 83 bpm (1,500 mm·min⁻¹ ÷ cardiac cycles).

The 6-s tracing shows 7.75 cardiac cycles; this computes to a heart rate of approximately 78 bpm (7.75 beats × 10).

The 1-minute ECG tracing displayed 80 bpm, so the 6-s tracing was a good method to use to determine this person's heart rate. Depending on which two cardiac cycles you chose, counting the distance between two consecutive cycles may not be a valid method of determining actual heart rate.

Measurement of VO$_{2max}$

33. The VO$_2$ (L/min) of a person walking who has a V$_I$ equal to 38.5 L/min, a V$_E$ equal to 37.3 L/min, and an F$_E$O$_2$ of 0.1695 would be (assuming a STPD correction factor of 0.7509):

$$VO_2 = (V_I \times F_IO_2) - (V_E \times F_EO_2)$$
$$VO_2 = (38.5 \text{ L/min} \times 0.2094) - (37.3 \text{ L/min} \times 0.1695)$$
$$VO_2 = (8.06 \text{ L/min}) - (6.32 \text{ L/min}) = 1.74 \text{ L/min}$$
$$VO_2 = 1.74 \text{ L/min} \times 0.7509 = 1.306 \text{ L/min}$$

34. The maximum MET score for this male athlete, who has an VO$_{2max}$ of 58.7 ml·kg⁻¹·min⁻¹ would be

Maximum MET = 58.7 ml·kg⁻¹·min⁻¹ × 1 MET/3.5 ml·kg⁻¹·min⁻¹ = 16.77 METs

35. The person's VO$_2$max is 55 ml·kg⁻¹·min⁻¹. If the person weighed 75 kg, then the absolute VO$_{2max}$ would be calculated as:

55 ml·kg⁻¹·min⁻¹ × 75 kg × 1 L/1000 ml
= 4.12 L·min⁻¹

36. If the person on the bicycle were consuming oxygen at a rate of 2.5 L·min⁻¹ and had a kcal to oxygen equivalent of 4.90 kcal·L⁻¹, then 60 minutes of exercise would result in an energy expenditure of:

2.5 L·min⁻¹ × 4.90 kcal·L⁻¹ × 60 min = 735 kcal

37. If the person's VO$_{2max}$ were 60 ml·kg⁻¹·min⁻¹ and he or she typically trains at 45 ml·kg⁻¹·min⁻¹, then the training intensity would be:

$$\frac{45 \text{ ml·kg}^{-1} \cdot \text{min}^{-1}}{60 \text{ ml·kg}^{-1} \cdot \text{min}^{-1}} = 75\%$$

Pulmonary Function

38. A spirogram indicates that a male subject has a VC of 4,800 ml. Assuming a BTPS correction factor of 1.11, what would be his actual VC (within the lungs)?

$$VC_{BTPS} = 4{,}800 \text{ ml} \times 1.11 = 5{,}328.0 \text{ ml}$$

39. Total lung capacity (TLC) is the summation of inspiratory reserve volume, tidal volume, expiratory reserve volume, and residual volume. Therefore, TLC is:

$$2000 \text{ ml} + 450 \text{ ml} + 1000 \text{ ml} + 900 \text{ ml}$$
$$= 4350 \text{ ml} = 4.35 \text{ L}$$

40. Forced expiratory volume (FEV) is that volume of air, expressed as a percentage of vital capacity, that can forcefully be expired in 1 second or 3 seconds. A very low FEV would suggest some sort of obstruction in the air passageways or very weak abdominal or intercostal muscles. FEV is calculated simply by dividing the expired volume by the vital capacity.

$$FEV_{1.0} = 4{,}480 \text{ ml} \div 5{,}600 \text{ ml} = 80\%$$

$$FEV_{3.0} = 5{,}490 \text{ ml} \div 5{,}600 \text{ ml} = 98\%$$

41. Use the appropriate equation to predict this person's vital capacity. First, convert height to cm by multiplying 72 inches by 2.54 cm·in^{-1}.

$$VC_{BTPS} \text{ (ml)} = [27.63 - (0.112 \times \text{age})] \times \text{height;cm}$$

$$VC_{BTPS} \text{ (ml)} = [27.63 - (0.112 \times 25)] \times 182.88 =$$

$$VC_{BTPS} \text{ (ml)} = [24.83] \times 182.88 = 4{,}540.9 \text{ ml}$$

Since the observed VC is equal to 5.0 L, the prediction equation underestimates the actual VC for this man by 459.1 ml.

42. Residual lung volume is a very important measurement for valid underwater weighing measurements. If equipment is unavailable to actually measure residual volume, prediction equations can be used. When prediction equations generate inaccurate individual results, body composition results may be greatly affected.

Females:

$$RV \text{ (L)} = 0.009 \text{ (age)} + 0.08128 \text{ (height; inches)} - 3.90$$
$$\text{Predicted RV} = 0.009 \text{ (24)} + 0.08128 \text{ (66 in)} -$$
$$3.90 = 1.68 \text{ L}$$

This prediction equation overestimates this woman's actual RV by 180 ml, which result in her percent fat being underestimated by about 2% body fat. Thus, it would be best to use the measured RV data to minimize error.

Appendix E
Sources for Equipment

Equipment needed for the various laboratory experiences may be purchased from the following vendors. The list is not all-inclusive; however, it may provide some guidance in finding suitable equipment.

Product	Manufacturer's Address
Weight/Height Scale	Detecto Scale Co. Webb City, Missouri (800/641-2008)
Universal Gym machine weights	Kidde Box 1270 Cedar Rapids, Iowa 52406 (319/365-7561)
Free weights (dumbbells)	York Barbell Co. Box 1707 York, Pennsylvania 17405 (800/358-YORK)
Grip dynamometer	C.H. Stoelting Co. 424 North Homan Ave. Chicago, Illinois 60624
Sit and reach box	Creative Health Product 9135 General Court Plymouth, Michigan 48170 (800/742-4478)
Goniometer	J.A. Preston Co. 71 Fifth Ave. New York, New York 10003
Leighton Flexometer	Leighton Flexometer East 1321 55th Ave. Spokane, Washington 99203
Blood pressure equipment (sphygmomanometers and cuffs)	W. A. Baum Co. 602 Oak St. Copiague, New York 11726 (or local medical supply)
Electronic heart rate monitor	Polar CIC Inc. 1000 Shames Drive Westbury, New York 11590 (800/227-1314)
Step Bench	Kustom Built Athletic Equip. Spokane, Washington (509/534-4680)

Product	Manufacturer's Address
Cycle ergometer (Monark)	Quinton Instrument Co. 2121 Terry Ave. Seattle, Washington 98121 (800/426-0337)
Stop watch	Creative Health Product 9135 General Court Plymouth, Michigan 48170 (800/742-4478
Skinfold caliper (Harpenden)	Quinton Instrument Co. 2121 Terry Ave. Seattle, Washington 98121 (800/426-0337)
Measuring tape	Creative Health Product 9135 General Court Plymouth, Michigan 48170 (800/742-4478)
Natant hydrostatic weighing	Write authors (c/o Jim George) Department of Exercise Science and Physical Education Arizona State University Tempe, Arizona 85287-0701
Timing Pad (power test)	Creative Health Product 9135 General Court Plymouth, Michigan 48170 (800/742-4478)
Electrocardiography equipment	Quinton Instrument Co. 2121 Terry Ave. Seattle, Washington 98121 (800/426-0337)
VO_{2max} measurement equipment	Quinton Instrument Co. 2121 Terry Ave. Seattle, Washington 98121 (800/426-0337)

Index